DYSLEXIA:
Theory & Practice
of
Remedial Instruction

DYSLEXIA:
Theory & Practice
of
Remedial Instruction

DIANA BREWSTER CLARK

York Press/Parkton, Maryland

This book was manufactured in the United States of America. Typography by Brushwood Graphics, Inc., Baltimore, Maryland. Printing and binding by McNaughton & Gunn, Inc., Ann Arbor, Michigan. Cover design by Joseph Dieter, Jr.

Library of Congress Catalog Card Number 88-51242
ISBN 0-912752-17-3
ISBN 0-912752-16-5 (pbk)

Contents

Foreword

As the world progresses and as technology makes obsolete many of the basic skills that were earlier deemed essential, reading remains paramount. Before the typewriter, good penmanship—the possession of a script that was legible and attractive—was highly valued. Before the calculator, it was important to be able to do quick and accurate "mental arithmetic." It is difficult, however, to think of any technological development that will wipe out the need for basic literacy, since reading skill is the foundation for almost all later learning and since, in the last analysis, reading is thinking.

To learn to read is the most important task of the young child starting school and to fail at this task is a serious matter. It is no wonder that more research studies have been conducted and more instructional programs have been developed in the field of reading than in any other area of education. As with most educational endeavors, there have been many different approaches and many conflicting claims as to what is effective. More often than not, these claims have remained unsubstantiated, both in terms of theory and research evidence and in terms of direct evaluation of the teaching approaches themselves. Too often we have spent our efforts on promoting intellectual controversies among competing claims, marketing instructional programs as if they were soap, and forgetting the ultimate goal of improving children's performance.

We have long recognized that not all children acquire reading skill at the same rate. Indeed, some children never manage to develop the proficiency in reading that we have come to consider every person's birthright. As the concept of dyslexia has emerged, so have confusion and controversy, for it is a difficult concept. Not being able to learn to read is a complex, multifaceted problem, and we have far to go before we understand the problem fully and can deal with it in a completely satisfactory way.

But recently, genuine progress has been made in the study of dyslexia. Reliable research findings are emerging and are being incorporated into effective instructional programs. They are also being incorporated into the consciousness of the professionals in the field—the classroom teacher, the reading co-ordinator, the school principal, and all the others who have responsibility for making all children literate.

Diana Clark's book offers a wealth of valuable and readily applicable information from a sound scholarly perspective. There is a careful and thorough description of the various instructional approaches and the specific techniques that they use. There is, as well, a solid presentation of the theory and empirical research on which these programs are based. Dr. Clark has provided us here with a comprehensive, up-to-date, and insightful study of the field of dyslexia.

Joanna P. Williams, Ph.D.
Professor of Psychology and Education
Teachers College, Columbia University

Preface

This book is written primarily for teachers engaged in language arts instruction for dyslexic students: remedial reading specialists, special education teachers, and reading and language arts teachers who are required to adapt instruction for disabled readers in their classrooms. These practitioners undoubtedly have the greatest influence over the educational outcome of dyslexic children. The book is also intended for undergraduate and graduate students of education who plan to work with dyslexic children, for they are the practitioners of the future. Additionally, it is my hope that professionals who make educational planning decisions for dyslexic children will be among its readers: school administrators, psychologists, and counselors.

The book's primary purpose is to provide practical information on methods of instruction in reading, writing, and spelling for dyslexic students. It presents this information against a backdrop of current research findings related to dyslexia and its treatment in order that its readers will understand the theoretical rationale behind these methods and thereby be able to judge their relative value.

The need for such a book became apparent in light of an extensive review I undertook of the research on dyslexia, or developmental reading disorder, and methods of instruction designed to treat this disorder. Added to my experience as a reading disabilities specialist engaged in both practice and research, the review led to several important realizations. The first is that a cure for dyslexia does not lie "just around the corner." Despite the considerable knowledge we have acquired over the last fifty years about the nature of this disorder, a multitude of unanswered questions remain, many of which may not be satisfactorily answered in the near future. It is encouraging to know that rapidly advancing techniques of neuropsychological investigation are helping us to identify the biological underpinnings of dyslexia; however, it may be a long time before we learn how to utilize this knowledge effectively in treating the disorder.

A second realization is that most of us involved in reading disabilities research have tended to overlook the fact that understanding developmental reading disorder is dependent upon understanding the process of normal reading development. Our disregard may be due in part to the fact that the psychology of normal reading development has been a field of inquiry hardly more enlightened than our own. In the last decade, however, significant progress has been made in reading research, and many of the findings, as well as newer theories, have enormous relevance for the study of dyslexia.

Another realization is that the separation of reading education, special education, and remedial reading education into three ostensibly autonomous domains of instruction—the first two residing in schools, the third for the most part in the private sectors—has been extremely detrimental to dyslexic students, causing unnecessary confusion over their identification and treatment. Sharing and integrating ideas between these three, now separate, disciplines is essential if dyslexic students are ever to be served effectively.

A fourth realization is that over the last twenty years considerable effort has been directed toward developing remedial methods and programs for teaching reading, writing, and spelling to dyslexic students. Some of these instructional approaches have been in practice for a notable length of time, yet information about them has been poorly disseminated. The major impetus for writing this book was my growing awareness that teachers and other professionals who work with dyslexic students need to be better informed about existing instructional methods for these students.

The development of remedial practice cannot afford to wait for definitive pronouncements from the field of research. However, as the research reviewed indicated, we have available a significant amount of potentially useful data on the nature of the reading process, the acquisition of reading skills, the characteristics of disabled readers, and the instructional conditions that enhance their learning. This information needs now to be recognized, synthesized, and brought to bear on the problem of dyslexia. Knowledge thus derived can then be imparted to teachers and educational planners so that they will be able to evaluate not only existing instructional methods and programs for dyslexic students but also those that might be developed in the future. That is what this book is meant to accomplish.

The book is divided into three parts. Part I consists of two chapters. The first chapter presents recent theories on the psychology of reading and reading development, placing particular emphasis on the skills required for learning to read in an alphabetic system. Chapter 1 sets the stage for a discussion of dyslexia, a condition that impinges on the ability to learn to read in this system. Chapter 2 examines the nature of dyslexia, the attendant reading, writing, and spelling problems, and the deficits known, or presumed, to underlie these problems.

Part II centers on remedial instruction for dyslexic students. It begins with a chapter on effective teaching principles and instructional techniques. Each of the following chapters focuses on remedial instruction in a reading related skill area which is problematic for dyslexic students: phonological awareness, phonic knowledge, automatic word recognition, reading fluency, reading comprehension, spelling, composition, and handwriting. In addition, the reciprocal relationship between reading, writing, and spelling instruction is examined.

Part III is devoted to remedial programs designed to teach reading, writing, and spelling to dyslexic students. It also considers several reading programs which, though not designed specifically for dyslexic students, have potential application for them, inasmuch as they incorporate many of the instructional principles that these students require. In each case, information is provided on the program's theoretical rationale, its curriculum and instructional methodology, its teacher training requirements, and its effectiveness as evidenced by evaluation studies. The last chapter addresses issues related to planning a comprehensive reading curriculum for dyslexic students and takes into account instructional components not provided in existing remedial programs which should be included. It ends with an exhortation that teachers prepare themselves to take stronger leadership positions in the education of dyslexic students.

Acknowledgements

I am indebted to the Good Samaritan Foundation of Wilmington, Delaware which, through a generous grant to Teachers College, funded the research review that led to this book, and I am very grateful to Jeannette Fleischner for giving me the opportunity to be in the right place at the right time. I would like to express my appreciation to Pam Dusenberry for her invaluable help as my research assistant and to Judith Birsh, Lois Dreyer, Lynn Gelzheiser, and Joanna Williams for reading my manuscript and for offering encouragement and advice. To Margaret Jo Shepherd I owe especial thanks for sharing her enthusiasm, her knowledge, and her ideas; she has been an ongoing source of support throughout this project. My thanks go also to my publisher, Elinor Hartwig, whose good judgment and sensitivity made the publication of this book a surprisingly pleasant experience for me. Lastly, I would like to commend Martha and Henry Sherrill for their enlightened efforts to obtain effective remedial instruction for dyslexic students. In our mutual concern about the education of dyslexic children, I count all these people as true friends.

To Elise, Ashley, and Brewster

PART

I

Reading and Dyslexia

CHAPTER

1

Perspectives on Reading and Learning to Read

Reading, a tremendously complex skill, is relatively new in human development. It is a skill that is not acquired naturally, but must be taught. Although some children learn to read more easily than others, all children require reading instruction. An ongoing controversy in reading education has been over what form this instruction should take, or indeed whether there is one method of instruction suitable for all students. This controversy is far from settled; however, one approach to resolving it has been to examine the act of reading and attempt to identify its component subskills in order to determine those that must be taught. A second approach has been to look at how learners differ in their ability to acquire these skills and to consider what consequences these learner differences have for reading instruction. This chapter focuses on the first approach.

The psychology of reading has been under investigation since the beginning of this century, but in the last fifteen to twenty years significant studies have been made in this field. Combined efforts of reading educators and researchers from related disciplines (e.g., psychology, neurology, linguistics) have led to new perspectives on the act of reading and learning to read, several of which have contributed substantially to the understanding of reading disability. One such perspective views reading as an *information processing system*. It attempts to identify the psychological processes involved in the act of reading and to determine how they are coordinated. Another perspective stresses the phonological processing demands that the *English alphabet* places on readers, particularly on children learning to read. A third perspective focuses on reading as a *developing process*. Yet a fourth perspective emphasizes the contribution of the reader's *background knowledge* to the act of reading. Each of these perspectives is discussed below.

INFORMATION PROCESSING THEORIES OF READING

The main purpose of reading is to become informed, or to gain meaning from text, whether for educational or recreational purposes. Opinions vary over how this purpose is fulfilled. Viewing reading as an information processing system provokes questions about what subprocesses are involved, the order in which they occur, and the relative contribution of the various available information sources. One extremely important query, for example, concerns the extent to which meaning or print guides the reading act. Reading theorists have developed models, or theoretical representations of the reading process, to explain their points of view on these issues. Three distinctly different positions on the reading process are discussed below.

TOP-DOWN THEORY

Proponents of this theory of reading, led by Kenneth Goodman and Frank Smith, take a strong meaning-based position, maintaining that reading is primarily dependent upon the reader's intention, or purpose, for reading a text. Rather than reading every word, good readers sample, or select out, only the essential textual information for meeting this purpose (Goodman 1967; Smith 1978, 1979). They rely heavily on their acquired knowledge of the world and of conventional graphemic, syntactic, and semantic structures to hypothesize or predict the words to come and to confirm the sense of what they have read. Only when they find that the text does not make sense do they go back and focus on individual words or examine letters in words.

Goodman calls reading a "psycholinguistic guessing game." Both Goodman and Smith describe reading as a top-down procedure, moving from higher (cognitive) to lower (perceptual) order mental processes, that is to say, from the attachment of meaning or purpose for reading to the perception of visual cues in the text.

BOTTOM-UP THEORY

Diametrically opposed to the Goodman–Smith perspective on reading is the bottom-up perspective. This model describes reading as a hierarchical procedure which moves from processing the smallest bits of graphemic information, individual letters, to ever larger chunks of information and only attaches semantic meaning after words have been identified (LaBerge and Samuels 1974).

An important contribution of the bottom–up model is its emphasis on the subprocesses of the reading act and its contention that many of these subprocesses, such as letter and word identification, must become automatic in order for readers to be fluent. David LaBerge and S. Jay Samuels (1974), who were among the first investigators to focus on the attentional demands of reading, hypothesize a "limited capacity mechanism" in human information processing that controls the distribution of attentional resources. As they explain it, during execution of a complex skill such as reading, many component processes must be coordinated within a very short time; if none of these processes is carried out automatically, there will not be enough attention available to execute the reading act successfully.

INTERACTIVE THEORY

Bottom–up and top–down models represent extreme theoretical perspectives on the act of reading. Both describe reading as a series of sequentially ordered processes and are therefore referred to as *serial processing models*. In contrast, another view of reading holds that many of the component processes occur in parallel. David Rumelhart (1977), who originally proposed this theory, contends that readers simultaneously initiate word identification and predict meaning, and he maintains that these are reciprocal events. He cites four sources of knowledge that the good reader has available to help extract the message in the text: orthographic knowledge (knowledge of letters, sounds, and spelling patterns), lexical knowledge (knowledge of words), syntactic knowledge (knowledge of sentence patterns), and semantic knowledge (knowledge of meaning). Rumelhart believes that these four knowledge sources can be activated concurrently and that they operate reciprocally; he refers to his theory as an interactive model of the reading process.

WEIGHING THE MODELS

Goodman and Smith's top–down model has, in fact, been called into question by recent studies that demonstrate that proficient readers do not skip over words and phrases, nor do they rely only on context to gain information. Instead, they fixate on almost all words in text (Just and Carpenter 1980). Fluent readers are less reliant on context in processing textual information than poor readers because they are more adept at recognizing individual words within the text (Stanovich 1986b). Thus accurate word recognition indeed appears to be an essential component of proficient reading.

Speed of word identification has also been shown to be a major determinant of reading ability (Perfetti 1984; Stanovich 1980). Correlations as high as .80 have been demonstrated between the rate of context-free word recognition and reading comprehension (Stanovich, Cunningham, and Feeman 1984). The strength of this relationship seems to bear out the limited attentional capacity thesis of LaBerge and Samuels. Charles Perfetti (1984, 1985b), another leading reading theorist, offers a similar explanation for this relationship which he calls "verbal efficiency theory." The more automatic the ability to recognize individual words in reading text, the greater the resources available for comprehending text.

The interactive model has gained acceptance among some of the more prominent researchers in the field of reading who claim that serial processing models fail to hold up under study. According to Keith Stanovich (1980), bottom-up models are unable to explain the effects of context on reading speed that have been observed under experimental conditions; top-down models must be rejected for the reasons cited above. Interactive models, on the other hand, can account for concurrent influences at all levels of processing because, as he expresses it, " . . . higher-level processes constrain the alternatives of lower-level processes but are themselves constrained by lower-level analyses" (Stanovich 1980). By "lower-level" Stanovich is referring to orthographic (letter clusters) and graphemic (letters) features in words.

Stanovich emphasizes the potentially compensatory nature of these interacting processes and calls his own view of reading an interactive-compensatory model. The finding that readers with poor word recognition are more reliant on context than good readers is one example of such compensation. Stanovich's interactive-compensatory model, because it illustrates so well the trade-offs that can occur among the component subskills of reading, helps to explain individual differences in reading ability. It therefore has considerable appeal for those of us concerned with disabled readers. There is much similarity between this theory and Perfetti's verbal efficiency theory.

ACKNOWLEDGING THE CHALLENGES OF THE ALPHABETIC SYSTEM

The abstract nature of our alphabet imposes unique demands on readers, particularly on students learning to read. In contrast to logographic writing systems, such as Chinese, where pictures or written symbols correspond to specific ideas or concepts, in alphabetic systems letters (graphemes) have no semantic import in and of themselves. Instead, they correspond to speech *sounds* (phonemes) which carry meaning only when blended together. As one reading expert put it, "the units of print map onto units of speech rather than units of meaning" (Perfetti 1984). In this abstract system, the learner must discover the alphabetic principle and master the phonetic code in order to become a truly competent reader.

The major advantage of our alphabet is its remarkable efficiency: with only twenty-six symbols, the writer of English can produce an uncalculable number of words. Furthermore, knowing the phonetic code makes possible the reading and writing of words never seen before (Perfetti 1984). For the learner, however, two basic features of the alphabet create significant challenges. The first is the fact that phonemes, particularly consonants, are abstractions. Phonemes only approximate speech sounds. They are not discrete elements that can be isolated within the speech stream. One cannot pronounce the consonant *b,* for example, without producing a schwa sound (e.g., "buh"). This feature makes it difficult not only for teachers to demonstrate letter sounds in isolation but also for students to distinguish them in the context of words. The second characteristic of the English alphabet that challenges the learner is the lack of individual letters to represent each vowel sound. The letter *a,* for example, stands for several different sounds (e.g., "cat," "cake," "call," "card") (Perfetti 1984).

Although most experts believe that good readers have acquired a large repertoire of familiar words which they can recognize automatically without phonological mediation, in other words, whose meanings they can obtain directly from print (Backman et al. 1984; Haines and Leong 1983; LaBerge 1979; Perfetti 1984, 1985b; Stanovich, Cunningham, and Cramer 1984), some respected theorists maintain that phonological processing occurs at all levels of reading (Liberman 1984; Pennington et al. 1987). According to Isabelle Liberman, the leading proponent of this thesis, linguistic information is stored in memory in its phonological form; therefore all word recognition requires letter sound access, or phonological recoding, which may be more or less apparent depending upon the level of reading fluency. Evidence that good readers have more difficulty remembering lists of visually presented words or letters that rhyme (e.g., *B, C, D*) than groups of items that are not phonetically confusable provides some support for Liberman's contention. Regardless of this controversy, phonological knowledge is essential for decoding words that are not yet familiar. The assumption that both phonological and visual means of word recognition are used alternatively, depending upon need, is usually referred to as the "dual access hypothesis."

PHONOLOGICAL AWARENESS

In the last decade, there has been increasing interest in children's phonological or linguistic awareness and how this awareness affects their ability to learn to read. Many reading authorities feel that a minimal level of understanding about the phonological aspects of language is a prerequisite for reading, particularly for reading an alphabetic orthography (Mattingly 1972). Agreement has not yet been reached on just what specific skills this level represents; however, such skills as the ability to recognize and create rhyme and the ability to identify initial sounds in spoken words or the number of syllables or phonemes in spoken words have been considered. For example, Lynette Bradley and Peter Bryant (1985), working in England, found that prereaders' sensitivity to rhyme and alliteration (ability to identify the initial letter) in orally presented words correlated significantly with later reading achievement. Tasks that require phonological analysis, such as asking children to say only part of a particular word (Fox and Routh 1980, 1983; Rosner 1974; Rosner and Simon 1971), have successfully identified children having difficulty learning to read.

More than ten types of phonological awareness tasks have been specified; however, in order to use them reliably to predict or identify reading problems, the sequence in which phonological skills are normally acquired, or their relative levels of difficulty, must be determined (Lewkowicz 1980; Stanovich, Cunningham, and Cramer 1984). We now know that distinguishing the boundaries of linguistic elements within the sound stream, also referred to as phonological segmentation, follows a developmental trend from larger to smaller linguistic units: first words in sentences, then syllables in words, and finally phonemes in syllables (Liberman et al. 1977; Fox and Routh 1980). When Liberman and her colleagues (Liberman et al. 1977) asked children to tap out the number of sounds they heard in words, most five year olds were able to segment by syllables but only a small percentage could do so by phonemes, and only 70 percent of six year olds were able to segment by phonemes. The fact that by second grade those children who could not segment phonemically as six year olds were performing at the bottom of their class in reading is one of many research findings indicating a significant relationship between phonemic segmentation ability and learning to read.

Despite the substantial evidence that phonological awareness and reading ability are related, it is not yet known whether the relationship is causal or reciprocal. In support of a causal relationship, Bradley and Bryant (1983, 1985) were able to demonstrate clear-cut effects of phonological analysis training on reading and spelling. They taught six- and seven-year-old children to group one-syllable words (represented by pictures) according to common sounds and to identify those sounds. At the end of the two year training period these children were reading and spelling several months ahead of children in a control group who had been taught to categorize words according to concepts. These results strongly suggest a causal relationship between at least one kind of phonological awareness— sound categorization—and reading. On the other hand, efforts to teach segmenting and blending skills to kindergarten children have not yielded demonstrable facilitative effects to date on later word reading ability (Fox and Routh 1984), and questions remain as to whether segmenting and particularly blending skills can actually be taught, whether most kindergarten children are ready to learn them or whether they are actually prerequisites for beginning reading.

Is the relationship between phonological awareness and learning to read reciprocal or causal? Linnea Ehri (1979, 1985), Anthony Jorm and David Share (1983), and other reading researchers argue that the relationship is reciprocal. Ehri believes that the awareness of print as language helps children to develop "linguistic insight," that "word consciousness" comes from experience in matching speech to print. An often cited study (Morais et al. 1979), in which adult illiterates were found to be significantly less aware of the phonological aspects of language than adults who had only recently learned to read, lends support to this position. The relationship between phonological awareness and reading apparently can be both causal and reciprocal. Young children who have developed these phonological skills are quicker to grasp the alphabetic principle. At the same time, exposure to print, the growing realization that written words correspond to spoken words, and the experience of learning to recognize those words (which usually begins with matching initial letters with initial sounds) helps most children to become cognizant of the phonological elements in words.

DEVELOPMENTAL PERSPECTIVES ON READING

In addition to studying the act of reading, as teachers we have much to learn from examining the process of learning to read. We must be ever mindful that reading at proficient levels and reading as a developing skill are quite different behaviors, and we must try to understand how they differ.

Reading is learned over many years, and for most people important changes in reading behavior occur over this span of time (Chall 1983b). Some of the most significant changes take place in the beginning years, as Andrew Biemiller (1970) observed in his year-long study of first graders learning to read. Analyzing oral reading errors of these beginning readers, Biemiller identifies three distinct acquisition phases: a first phase marked by semantically or syntactically acceptable substitution errors, indicating that children are relying on contextual information for reading unfamiliar words; a second phase where the predominant errors are nonresponses and graphically similar word substitutions (e.g., "horse" for "house"), showing that they are attending to the graphic features of words; and a third phase involving both contextually and graphically constrained errors which Biemiller considers evidence that children are using both graphic and contextual information for reading new words.

Jeanne Chall (1983b), one of the leading researchers in reading education in this country, has developed a stage theory of reading development, which she prefers to call a scheme or model. She hypothesizes six qualitatively different stages from readiness to maturity. She maintains that most people progress through these stages in the same order, though not necessarily at the same rate, and despite the fact that many people do not reach the higher stages, or expert levels, of reading ability. She believes that rate and success in learning to read are determined by the interaction between learner and environment. Borrowing from Jean Piaget's stage theory of cognitive development (Inhelder and Piaget 1958; Piaget 1970), Chall describes reading as "a form of problem solving in which readers adapt to their environment through the processes of assimilation and accommodation" (1983b). Assimilation refers to the learner's application of previously acquired skills to a particular task or problem. Accommodation refers to the learner's ability to adopt new skills or new ways of thinking in performing an unfamiliar task or solving a new problem.

Chall provides ages and grade levels at which the average student may be expected to reach each of the six stages, but urges that they be considered only approximations. The longest stage in Chall's model is Stage 0, the prereading stage, lasting from birth to age six and comprising a greater amount of developmental change than any other stage. This period includes the very beginnings of an individual's language awareness to the ability (in the case of many preschool children) to recognize and name letters of the alphabet and even to read some popular names on signs and packages or some words in familiar books. Readiness concepts such as understanding the purpose of reading, understanding the relationship between pictures and print, understanding the relationship between written and spoken words, being able to rhyme, to alliterate (match initial sounds), and to segment units of speech (words in sentences and syllables in words, if not phonemes in words) are some of the readiness concepts acquired by most children during this stage. The end of this stage corresponds to Biemiller's first phase of reading acquisition in which children rely on memory for story content and other contextual strategies to guess at words. At this point, as Chall puts it, children bring more to the printed page than they take out.

Stage 1, the initial or decoding stage, is attained by most children between the ages of six and seven while in first and second grade. The major accomplishment of this period is grasping the alphabetic principle and learning the letter-sound correspondences, or the alphabetic code. This stage corresponds to Biemiller's second phase of reading acquisition in which children increasingly attend to graphic elements in words rather than treating words as wholes. Chall explains the successful transition from Stage 0 to Stage 1 as a process of accommodation: Children apply their newly acquired readiness concepts and skills, which include the ability to analyze parts within wholes, to the challenge of reading unfamiliar words. However, if these readiness skills are lacking, children approach new challenges through assimilation, continuing to use the strategies learned in the previous stage: viewing all words holistically and relying on contextual cues such as pictures and memory for stories.

Stage 2 involves confirming what has been learned in the previous stage and gaining fluency. It corresponds to Biemiller's third stage of reading acquisition in which children integrate both graphic and contextual information in reading words. Although their knowledge of phonics continues to develop during this period and even later, through extensive practice with reading material having familiar content, children gain confidence in applying "their decoding knowledge, the redundancies of the language, and the redundancies of the stories" (Chall 1983b). They begin to develop speed as well as accuracy in word recognition. At this point, the learner should be attending to both meaning and print and using cues from these information sources interactively. Stage 2 is a particularly critical period for the developing reader; if progress breaks down, the individual can remain "glued to print," as Chall expresses it. Many factors may contribute to this arrest, among them unstable phonic knowledge, limited experience with language and ideas, and lack of reading practice.

Stage 3, which commences in fourth grade at roughly nine years of age, is primarily distinguished from the previous stage by a change in motivation for reading. At this point, the individual begins to read in order to learn new information. Content area subjects (science and social studies) are introduced in school. Vocabulary enlargement and expansion of world knowledge become increasingly important. For the most part, the material encountered during this stage presents only one point of view. However, in the second half of Stage 3 (grades seven through eight or nine) which covers junior high, as students begin to read newspapers, magazines, and more adult materials, they are exposed to differing points of view and begin to read critically.

The ability to deal with multiple viewpoints is more fully developed in Stage 4 (ages fourteen through eighteen) which covers the high school years. This ability is acquired mainly through formal education.

Readers who attain the highest level of reading development, Stage 5, have learned to read selectively and are able to develop their own opinions and make their own judgments about what they read. As Chall expresses it, the reading process at this stage is "essentially constructive"; readers construct their own knowledge from that of others. Stage 5 is not usually reached until college age or later and may, in fact, be reserved for individuals who have an intellectual bent; Chall points out that four years of college does not ensure its attainment. It has not yet been determined what proportion of the general population become expert readers.

Each stage builds on the skills acquired in previous stages, and success in meeting the challenges confronted at each stage is to a large extent dependent upon mastery of those skills normally acquired in earlier stages, according to Chall. As they progress to higher stages, readers become increasingly flexible in their reading style, able to adjust the pace and the distribution of attention as the complexity of the material and the purpose for reading warrants. Under different conditions, bottom–up or top–down processes may dominate alternatively, or they may be more or less in balance. For example, in order to decode unfamiliar technical words, readers even at Stage 5 may resort to bottom–up processing, calling to use the phonic skills they learned in Stage 1. On the other hand, when searching a text for particular facts or skimming to get the gist of a text, top-down processes predominate.

In providing a conceptual framework for viewing reading acquisition, Chall's model of reading development contributes significantly to the understanding of reading problems. We need to keep in mind, however, that this is only a theory; we should be especially prudent about its practical application. As with all developmental models, there is a danger that the developmental milestones may be regarded too rigidly.

THE ROLE OF BACKGROUND KNOWLEDGE

Another way to look at reading is from the point of view of the reader's accumulated store of information and its influence on the ability to process text. Theoretically, all knowledge that the reader brings to bear on the process of reading and learning to read can be considered part of this background store (graphemic, phonological, orthographic, syntactic, and semantic). However, reading researchers and educators who stress the importance of background knowledge have been primarily concerned with semantic knowledge, or knowledge of the world, and its contribution to the comprehension of text. This perspective relates in some respects to top-down theory, because it views reading as a constructive process and emphasizes the role that the reader's familiarity with the subject matter in a text plays in comprehension or interpretation of that text.

Theorists have proposed that prior knowledge is stored in memory in the form of schemata (Anderson 1977; Rumelhart 1980; Thorndyke and Hayes-Roth 1979). Schemata can be thought of as psychological frameworks representing various generic concepts, as, for instance, "school," "restaurant," "breakfast"; they are essentially prototypes of meaning underlying these concepts (Rumelhart 1980). When applied to reading comprehension, schemata can be viewed as presuppositions about the meaning of the text (Eckwall and Shanker 1983). Experimental studies support schema theory by showing the effects of readers' background knowledge on their interpretation of text. In one such study, two passages about a wedding, one an American ceremony, the other Indian, were presented to both American and Indian subjects; American subjects understood and remembered more about the American wedding and vice versa (Steffenson, Joag-Dev, and Anderson 1979).

Although in this example schemata seem to have worked only in a top-down direction, they should not be construed as immutable. Ideally, schemata are able to accommodate to new experiences and new information and thus are constantly changing or developing. In this respect, the relationship between the reader's background knowledge and the text can be viewed as interactive. It can also be viewed as reciprocal, for just as the reader's background knowledge facilitates comprehension of text, extensive experience with text (reading) increases and enhances background knowledge.

EDUCATIONAL IMPLICATIONS OF DIFFERING PERSPECTIVES ON READING
READING INSTRUCTION

Not all reading authorities agree that knowing the phonetic code is essential for learning to read, nor do they acknowledge to the same extent the inherent challenges of the alphabetic system. Perspectives on these issues have important implications for reading instruction. Theorists who espouse a strong meaning-based or top-down view of reading tend to minimize the importance of learning the phonetic code. They believe that phonological knowledge should be called on in decoding unfamiliar words only as a last resort, that is, after all visual, semantic, and syntactic cues have failed. Proponents of this view advocate a visual approach to reading instruction that begins with teaching whole words rather than individual letter sounds. The choice of words to be taught is usually based on their frequency of use in students' environments. Phonetic regularity is not an important consideration; in fact, a large proportion of the most frequently used words in English are not phonetically regular (e.g., was, said, were) (Chall 1983a). This approach to reading instruction is generally referred to as the *whole-word* or *look-say* method. It is the method found in the more traditional basal reader programs.

In direct contrast to the whole-word or meaning-based method of beginning reading instruction is the *phonics-first* or *code-emphasis approach* advocated by reading experts who stress the phonological aspects of the alphabet and the demands that the alphabetic principle places on readers. This approach begins with teaching individual letter sounds that are then blended into words. Phonic elements are presented in a prescribed sequence, and each skill is directly taught. Practice in reading text involves only words that are phonetically spelled and that contain the letter sounds that have been taught, the exception being essential noncontent words that do not conform to phonetic spelling rules (e.g., is, was, said). Thus the vocabulary in beginning phonics readers is even more restricted than that of conventional basal readers. This method is also referred to as the *synthetic phonics approach*.

Somewhere in between these two extreme approaches to reading instruction lie most of the reading programs used in this country today. The majority of the newer basal programs do include some form of phonics instruction while still emphasizing a meaning-based, whole-word approach to reading. However, Jeanne Chall (1983a) observes in her analysis of existing beginning reading programs that phonics instruction in most basal programs is provided nonsystematically in follow-up activities and often not coordinated with the stories to be read. For these reasons, some teachers may opt to omit phonics instruction altogether from their reading lessons. It is assumed that children placed in these basal reading programs will automatically learn phonics generalizations from exposure to the whole words being taught, by becoming aware of sounds within these words and noting similarities in letter patterns between words having the same sounds. This method has been called *intrinsic phonics* or the *analytical phonics approach*.

After examining the relevant research studies, Chall (1983a) concludes that earlier and more intensive phonics instruction produces greater gains in reading by third grade. She finds convincing evidence that direct, systematic phonics instruction (the synthetic approach) is significantly more effective than the indirect, intrinsic or analytical approach.

READINESS INSTRUCTION

None of the existing reading programs designed for regular classroom use stresses the development of phonological awareness or teaches it systematically. Yet many basal programs include readiness workbooks that provide practice in identifying initial sounds in words represented by pictures or matching pictured items that rhyme, essentially phonological skills. Most readiness workbooks give practice in identifying initial letters in words, which is one form of phonemic segmentation. Only one published program, the Lindamood Auditory Discrimination in Depth, deals systematically with phonological segmentation. This program, which has been adopted in a few school districts as a preventive measure, was originally designed for remedial instruction in clinical settings, and is discussed in Chapter 13.

RELEVANCE OF READING STAGES TO GRADE ORGANIZATION

Chall (1983b) observes that her hypothetical stages of reading development parallel the organization of grades within schools. A particularly salient example of this parallel is the transition from Stage 2 to Stage 3, expected to occur around the beginning of fourth grade, which for a long time has been recognized as a pivotal point in children's educational lives. The radically new demands on students as they move into content area subjects—reading mainly now to gain information rather than just to improve their reading ability, dealing usually for the first time with expository text, encountering extensive amounts of new vocabulary—place many of them in jeopardy. Failure to master the skills normally acquired in earlier stages is a frequent cause of their unpreparedness for meeting these challenges.

These requisite skills include decoding, the ability to decipher unfamiliar words by analyzing their phonological (letter-sound) features and orthographic (spelling) patterns; fluency, automatic recognition of a large number of words and the ability to read these words in connected discourse; and comprehension, the ability to understand the meaning of the text. The development of proficient reading comprehension, which is now critical for success in school, may be delayed not only by poor decoding skills and lack of fluency, but also by insufficient background knowledge. The expansion of background knowledge itself may be adversely affected by limited reading experience, an example of the reciprocal nature of the reading development process. Chall (1983b) points out that as preparation for the transition to fourth grade, children need extensive reading practice with a wide variety of reading materials. It is not surprising that this is the point at which dyslexic students are often identified.

SUMMARY

The research-based perspectives on reading and learning to read and their implications for reading instruction presented here provide a background for a discussion of dyslexia, or specific reading disability. These perspectives include: (1) theories on the reading process, emphasizing an interactive relationship between reader, environment, and text; (2) recognition of the phonological demands which the alphabetic system places on readers, particularly on learners; (3) analysis of reading development as a series of stages which are marked by differing behaviors but build incrementally on each other; and (4) appreciation of the influential role of background knowledge in the reading process and the reciprocal relationship between background knowledge and reading development.

I believe that awareness of the complexity of the reading process and the challenges involved in learning to read, in addition to knowledge of how reading is generally taught in schools, will help us to understand dyslexia and the instructional needs of dyslexic students.

CHAPTER
2

The Nature of Dyslexia

TOWARD A DEFINITION

Before discussing the problem of dyslexia and its treatment, it is necessary to define or clarify the problem. A unanimously acceptable definition for dyslexia has not yet been formulated. In fact, there has probably been as much controversy over how to define this disorder as over how to treat it. The term itself derives from the Greek morphs *dys* (difficult) and *lexicos* (pertaining to words) and was first used by Berlin in 1887 to define a unique form of learning disorder characterized by extreme difficulty learning to read and spell words, despite conventional instruction. The disorder is thought to result from specific brain dysfunction in processing written language (Bryant 1985), though the origin and precise location of this dysfunction remain as yet unverified.

Dyslexia is not attributable to subnormal intelligence or socioeconomic deprivation nor to physical, sensory, or emotional handicaps, though it may coexist with any of these factors. Because the syndrome is easily confounded with reading problems caused by other deterimental circumstances, most of the numerous definitions of dyslexia contain exclusionary clauses stating what dyslexia is not. The fact that these clauses are often more extensive than the information provided on known characteristics of the disorder has led to the criticism that dyslexia has been arbitrarily defined as a "residual disorder," that is, "What is left after everything else is accounted for," (Inouye and Sorenson 1985) or as a middle-class disease. While they may help in identifying dyslexia, definitions by exclusion add little to our knowledge of how to treat dyslexia.

Dyslexia has also been referred to as *specific or developmental reading disability.* The qualifier "specific" is intended to connote a syndrome distinct from other types of reading disabilities, presumably those deriving from any of the extenuating conditions mentioned above. The word "developmental" refers to a disorder of suspected congenital or hereditary origin, in contrast to acquired dyslexia, a disorder resulting from brain injury occurring after the onset of reading (Frith 1986).[1] It is important to state that use of the term "developmental" does not mean that the disorder disappears with maturity. A distinguishing characteristic of dyslexia is, in fact, its persistence, although appropriate remedial treatment and the development of compensatory strategies may moderate its effects. In the last twenty years the terms "dyslexia" and "learning disabilities" have come to be used almost interchangeably even though the latter classification theoretically encompasses a broader range of cognitive deficits, such as math or attention deficits. The term "learning disabilities" actually has no inherent meaning but is rather a political label which was adopted to acquire special services for students with mild learning handicaps who did not qualify for placement in previously established special education categories—mentally handicapped, emotionally handicapped, physically handicapped, and so on. Although the large majority of students who are classified as learning disabled have reading difficulties, in many cases these difficulties can be attributed to mildly handicapping factors or conditions other than dyslexia, such as low average intelligence. Admittedly, the adoption of the learning disabilities classification has provided special instruction for many students whose educational needs were not being served in regular classrooms, but it has added further confusion and delay to the establishment of an operable definition of dyslexia and to the identification of dyslexic individuals. A large proportion of the research aimed at investigating dyslexia has used subjects classified as learning disabled, and therefore the validity of the results, as they relate to dyslexia, are open to question.

Throughout this book studies using subjects referred to as "reading disabled" are cited where the behavioral characteristics of these subjects resemble those of dyslexic individuals. However, it is important to note that the term reading disability does not imply a neurological basis for the manifested problems as do the classifications dyslexia and learning disabilities.

Because the neurological anomalies that distinguish dyslexia from

---

[1]Dyslexia is described under the heading "Developmental Reading Disorder" in the most recent revision of the *Diagnostic and Statistical Manual of Mental Disorders (DSM III)*, published by the American Psychiatric Association.

other forms of reading disability are extremely elusive, and because there is not yet a clear, concise, yet comprehensive, definition of the disorder, the best way to understand dyslexia is to examine the learning difficulties associated with the syndrome. Some of these learning difficulties are experienced by all dyslexic individuals and can therefore be considered major characteristics of dyslexia, even though they may differ in type and severity and may be more or less evident. Other learning-related deficits that I will discuss appear to be experienced by some, but not all, dyslexics. Such variation in symptoms provokes the question: Is dyslexia a unitary disorder or are there subtypes within the syndrome? This question will be addressed later in this chapter.

MANIFESTATIONS OF DYSLEXIA
READING PROBLEMS

Dyslexia is generally perceived first and foremost as a reading disorder. However, we are only just beginning to understand the specific nature of this disorder. It is necesssary to investigate the performance of dyslexic individuals on the various subskills required for proficient reading in order to determine where the problems occur. Deficits in the areas of word decoding, phonological analysis, automatic word recognition, use of context, and comprehension of text have all been observed in dyslexic readers.

Decoding Problems. The most pronounced among the number of reading difficulties that dyslexics experience is the inability to decode unfamiliar words (Olson et al. 1985; Siegel 1985; Vellutino 1983). This problem appears to be the common denominator in all cases of dyslexia (Gough and Tumner 1986). Furthermore, follow-up studies of dyslexic individuals indicate that the problem persists throughout schooling and adulthood (Aaron and Philips 1986; Forrell and Hood 1985; Frauenheim and Heckerl 1983; Read and Ruyter 1985).

The basis for the decoding deficiencies among dyslexic readers is their incomplete mastery of letter-sound correspondences that would help them articulate written words not automatically recognized. Dyslexic readers evidence extreme difficulty grasping the alphabetic principle and learning the phonetic code, knowledge essential to successful reading in an alphabetic system. They have trouble breaking down words in order to identify their component parts and in blending together these parts once they have been identified to pronounce written words. Sound sequencing errors (articulating letter sounds in the wrong order), as well as letter-sound confusions (producing the wrong sound for a given letter or letters), are often observed in their oral reading. Sometimes their letter-sound substitution errors appear to reflect reversals or transpositions of the written stimuli (e.g., /d/ for *b;* /p/ for *b;* "was" for "saw").

The adverse effects of their insecure grapheme-phoneme knowledge is particularly apparent when dyslexic readers are asked to decode nonsense words. In fact, this task, although artificial, has proven to be the most sensitive identifier of disabled readers (Read and Ruyter 1985; Richardson, DiBenedetto, and Adler 1982; Siegel 1985; Ryan, Miller, and Witt 1984). It has therefore been included in several assessment batteries aimed at diagnosing reading difficulties, such as the recently developed Decoding Skills Test (Richardson and DiBenedetto 1985).

Word Recognition Problems.   Dyslexics are slower and less accurate at identifying words that should be familiar to them. This problem is most evident with words presented in isolation (Perfetti 1984; Stanovich 1980). It may be less obvious when they are reading connected text and are able to use the context to help compensate, but when even the words in the surrounding context cannot be recognized automatically, their reading is severely impaired.

As discussed in Chapter 1, lack of reading accuracy and automatic recognition at the word level appears to place limitations on the comprehension of text, as well as on reading fluency (Stanovich, Cunningham, and Feeman 1984). David LaBerge and S. Jay Samuels (1974) attempted to explain this apparent trade off in attentional resources by hypothesizing a limited capacity mechanism in working memory. In the same vein, Charles Perfetti (1984, 1985b) proposes a verbal efficiency mechanism to account for the strong relationship between speed and accuracy of word identification and reading comprehension shown in correlational studies.

Inefficient Use of Context.   Although dyslexic readers are more reliant on context than are good readers in processing information in text, their efficiency in utilizing the context is limited by their relative lack of fluency in processing the context itself. A teacher or clinician working with dyslexic students will observe differing treatment of context among dyslexic students, depending upon personality as well as ability level. At one extreme, there may be the seemingly impulsive student whose word reading errors indicate gross misinterpretation of the surrounding context. At the other extreme, there may be the overly cautious word-by-word reader who simply comes to a halt when unable to recognize a word, either because of hesitancy to venture a guess or because decoding efforts and/or slow reading pace prevents the reader from remembering what he or she has read.

Reading Comprehension Problems.   Not surprisingly, dyslexic readers as a group have poorer reading comprehension than good readers. Although comprehension problems are usually less conspicuous than decoding difficulties, in classroom settings where oral reading requirements are minimal, dyslexia may only be picked up on standardized tests of reading comprehension. Such tests are usually not administered until third grade or later. Indeed, some bright dyslexic students are able to mask their reading disability through compensation for many years. Among the most gifted dyslexic students, there are cases where the deleterious effects of the disability surface only on the college entrance examinations, where they are presented with long passages of highly sophisticated content to be read within strict time constraints. The evidence to date indicates that the greater portion of the poorer reading comprehension exhibited by dyslexics is explained by their slower and less accurate word reading (Perfetti 1985b; Stanovich 1986a). Time limits exacerbate the problem, as P. G. Aaron and Scott Philips (1986) discovered in examining the academic skills of dyslexic college students. From test administration, they find that the reading comprehension level of all the dyslexic subjects in their investigation is well above their reading speed level.

In some cases of dyslexia, however, factors other than decoding problems may be implicated in poor reading comprehension. For example, dyslexic children are found to have deficits in listening comprehension (Smiley et al. 1977) and difficulties understanding complex sentences in speech as well as reading (Byrne 1981; Vogel 1975). Where these problems exist, we do not yet know whether they are basic to or derivative of dyslexia. Extrinsic factors such as reading experience and academic instruction, as well as home environment, undoubtedly influence the development of syntax in normal children. At the same time, studies show young dyslexic children to be deficient, relative to normal age-matched children, in grammatical understanding and morphological knowledge (Byrne 1981; Menynuk and Flood 1981).

One explanation offered for the syntactic processing deficiencies exhibited by some dyslexic children is that they are due to phonological coding deficits. Support for this hypothesis comes in part from studies showing that the syntactic errors made by dyslexic children in sentence comprehension are different from those of normal children only in degree, not in kind (Mann, Shankweiler, and Smith 1984). Isabelle Liberman and her colleagues, who have led this line of research, maintain that as we read or listen we must hold incoming linguistic information in working memory in phonological form while we process sentences (e.g., Liberman and Shankweiler 1985). Bolstering their position is evidence from experimental studies showing that suppressing phonological coding interferes with sentence comprehension and most specifically with processing syntax (Abernathy, Martin, and Caramazza 1982; Kleiman 1975). It is suggested that dyslexic individuals not only have trouble learning the phonological code but also generating this code in order to maintain linguistic information in short-term, or working, memory while comprehending sentences (Brendt 1983; Liberman and Shankweiler 1985). These issues are discussed further in the section headed "Short-Term Verbal Memory Deficits" (see page 28).

Many dyslexics have particular difficulty processing function words, articles, conjunctions and other lexical items that serve to connect syntactic relations (Blank and Bruskin 1982). This problem may derive from phonological coding weaknesses; function words have little semantic meaning in and of themselves and therefore require a greater degree of phonological processing for maintenance in working memory than do content words (Brendt 1983). The frequent omissions and substitutions of inflectional morphemes made by dyslexics have also been attributed to phonological deficits (Aaron and Philips 1986). However, not all dyslexic children demonstrate serious deficits in syntax and morphology; the question arises whether those who do have these problems suffer from specific language impairment or whether those who do not have these problems have a less severe form of dyslexia.

Because of their general lack of reading experience many dyslexic individuals fail to develop a strong knowledge base, which further delimits their ability to comprehend and remember text material (Stanovich 1986b; Torgesen 1985). Insufficient background knowledge can be considered a secondary order comprehension problem. At the same time, some disabled readers, who might be judged dyslexic, seem to use background knowledge inappropriately. Katherine Maria and Walter MacGinitie (1982) have observed poor readers with high verbal IQ scores who tend to overrely on prior knowledge in processing written text. As they described it, these children

> . . . use a few words in the text to call up related background knowledge, but are not much constrained by the information in the text. They read as if the text is simply saying whatever it is that they already know. These children are assimilating the text to their schemata, but they are failing to accommodate. (Maria and MacGinitie 1982)

The children in the Maria and MacGinitie studies applied this overdependence on top-down processing, or "nonaccommodating" strategy, to their listening comprehension of text as well as to their reading comprehension; therefore, they cannot be compensating for poor word decoding skills only. Although these children apparently have no trouble comprehending oral language in everyday situations, they have difficulty processing written language, regardless of its presentation. Maria and MacGinitie call attention to the various elements of written language not typical of spoken language that seem to present problems for these children. These include greater lexical density (less redundancy) and more complex syntax. Processing written language, therefore, places greater demands on verbal short-term memory than does spoken language, which is one possible reason for the overreliance on background knowledge observed in these poor readers. Another plausible explanation is that although they may be able to mask their basic decoding deficit, these bright, verbal, dyslexic children have had limited experience with written language relative to their normal reading peers. They are less familiar with linguistic conventions, such as words that signal relationships between sentences and other elements in text. Many pay little attention to pronouns, conjunctions, adverbs marking time or place, or other words that serve as cohesive devices in text processing. This problem has been widely noted among disabled readers (e.g., Aaron and Philips 1986; Blank and Bruskin 1982). It is my feeling that both phonological processing deficiencies and lack of reading experience are responsible for the weaknesses in written language comprehension among dyslexic individuals.

SPELLING PROBLEMS

For dyslexic individuals, spelling presents even greater challenges than reading, and indeed this is probably so for most people. Margaret Stanback and Marylee Hansen, who undertook a comprehensive review of the research on spelling instruction, suggest that spelling difficulty "may be the single most common academic failing of learning disabled children" (Stanback and Hansen 1980). Not only do spelling deficits inevitably attend reading problems, these investigators maintain, but they are always the more severe of the two disabilities. Furthermore, among people who are dyslexic, spelling deficiencies persist into adulthood (Aaron and Philips 1986; Cone et al. 1985; Ganschow 1984; Rutter, 1978).

Stanback and Hansen cite three potential sources for the disproportionate difficulty of spelling and reading, the first being a *visual factor:* Spelling places greater demands on visual memory than does reading. The second suggested source is an *auditory factor:* Spelling often requires isolating speech sounds, which is more difficult than isolating letters in print, especially for young children. The third source is an *orthographic factor:* The unbalanced ratio of phonemes to letters or letter combinations representing these phonemes leaves a larger number of possible responses for the speller than for the reader.

Although we know that dyslexic persons have spelling problems, we are not as knowledgeable about the nature of these problems. In investigating spelling disorders in dyslexic individuals, much of the research relies on analyses of spelling errors. Elena Boder (1971), for example, claims to find three distinct spelling patterns among dyslexic individuals. She terms these error patterns dysphonetic (reflecting deficits in sound-symbol association), dyseidetic (representing difficulty remembering visual aspects of words with nonphonetic spellings), and dysphonetic-dyseidetic (a combination of both problems). In a random sample of 107 students diagnosed as dyslexic, Boder and Jarrico (1982) judged 63 percent to be dysphonetic, 10 percent to be dyseidetic, 23 percent dysphonetic-dyseidetic; the remaining 6 percent could not be classified. Attempts to substantiate the validity of Boder's spelling subtypes, however, have not been successful on the whole (Carpenter 1983; Moats 1983; Nockleby and Galbraith 1984).

Rebecca Treiman and Jonathan Baron (1983) examine spelling behaviors in dyslexic individuals from the perspective of rule application. They find evidence of dyslexics who are overly reliant on spelling-sound rules, whom they have labeled "Phoenecians," and a group who depend on word-specific associations, whom they call "Chinese." These investigators allege that the Phoenician type of dyslexic is able to spell nonsense words but tends to overgeneralize phonics rules to exception words.

Roderick Barron (1980) observes that poor readers are more likely to use a visual-orthographic strategy in reading and to apply a phonological strategy to spelling. Lynette Bradley and Peter Bryant find this same strategy differential in young normal readers (Bradley and Bryant 1979; Bradley 1985). They believe that the independence of reading and spelling behaviors is a natural developmental phenomenon: Young children who have not yet learned to read often spell words on the basis of sound.

Also investigating the dissociation between reading and spelling, Uta and Charles Frith (Frith and Frith 1983) propose a stage theory of strategy acquisition in the development of proficient spelling. In the first stage, the child learns to analyze speech sounds in spoken words. In the second stage, the child learns to convert speech sounds, or phonemes, into their written counterparts, or graphemes. In the third stage, which the Friths call the orthographic state, the child learns to select from among the phonetically plausible choices the graphemes which are conventionally correct in any particular spelling. In observing twelve-year-old children, the Friths have been able to identify three groups of readers: good readers-good spellers, poor readers-poor spellers, and good readers-poor spellers. They maintain that poor readers-poor spellers, having not mastered the phonetic code, make predominantly nonphonetic spelling errors and can be considered dyslexic. Good readers-poor spellers, on the other hand, have trouble remembering spellings that do not conform to phonological rules and tend to compensate by spelling all words phonetically; they have not reached the second stage nor learned orthographic conventions. In contrast, good readers who are also proficient spellers are able to apply visual-orthographic strategies to spelling as well as reading. How to account for the good readers-poor spellers is not clarified, though the Friths find evidence of subtle reading problems among this group. Whether good readers-poor spellers represent a type of dyslexia or a point on a continuum of language skill development is not yet known.

Michael Gerber and Robert Hall (1987) question the validity of the error analysis paradigm as applied to the research on spelling disorders; they point out the lack of an empirically supported basis for classifying errors as phonetic or nonphonetic. In addition, they criticize this approach for being too static and for failing to account for developmental change in spelling acquisition. They cite the earlier work of Charles Read (1975) who, in comparing the spelling of learning disabled students with that of younger normally achieving children, found similar error patterns. More recent studies also show error pattern likenesses between these groups (Bruck 1988; Carpenter 1983; Moats 1983).

Gerber and Hall propose an information processing model of spelling acquisition based on empirical observations of both novice spellers and learning disabled students. Their model describes the growth of speed and accuracy as learners gain mastery over the various component mechanisms involved in spelling, including phonemic analysis and segmentation, grapheme-phoneme association, pattern recognition, and so on. The dual nature of English spelling is taken into account as is the need for learners to acquire both lexical or word specific information, such as knowledge of morphemes, homophones, irregular patterns, and nonlexical or phonetic information, such as grapheme-phoneme relationships. Automaticity is arrived at through repeated experience in utilizing these two information sources to "systematically reduce uncertainty and facilitate orderly search and retrieval from long-term store," which they refer to as "controlled processing" (Gerber and Hall 1987). A major point made by these researchers is that dyslexic students do not seem to benefit from repeated exposure to "formal spelling instruction and word manipulation in school contexts" as do normally achieving students. At the same time, these investigators acknowledge that spelling instruction in most schools today is limited and of generally poor quality.

EXPRESSIVE WRITING PROBLEMS

Unfortunately, little research exists on the written expression problems of dyslexics. That which has been done pertains for the most part to adolescents, probably because writing problems exceed reading problems in this age group (King 1985; Ganschow 1984). Poor written expression is one of the major distinguishing characteristics of the adolescent dyslexic (Poplin et al. 1980). Since most reading activities in older school-age children are conducted silently, reading difficulties in undiagnosed dyslexics may go unnoted. In contrast, writing problems become more conspicuous with each school year as the writing demands in the curriculum increase.

When we consider the three potential areas of writing difficulties for dyslexic people—written formulation, spelling, and handwriting (Cicci 1983)—spelling stands out as by far the most prevalent deficit area (Ganschow 1984; Poplin et al. 1980). Other types of deficiencies can also be found in the writing samples of dyslexic students—for example, poor punctuation, word omissions, lack of subject/predicate number agree-ment, and lower percentages of compound and/or complex sentences—but as yet we have no consistent documentation of their prevalence. In a very recent study with learning disabled students, comparing stories that they dictated to an examiner with stories that they wrote by hand or on a word processor, dictated stories were significantly longer, of better qual-ity, and contained fewer grammatical errors. These findings suggest that, " . . . mechanical and conventional demands of producing text appear to interfere with the fluency and quality of written expression" (MacArthur and Graham 1988).

However, perhaps the most serious writing problem among peo-ple who are dyslexic and one that so many dyslexic students experience, is a general resistance to writing. As Diana King (1985), who works with dyslexic adolescents, affirms, without remedial intervention this resis-tance tends to build throughout the school years.

One of the major problems besetting the field of writing research has been a lack of adequate measurement procedures. At the present time, the two most frequently used standardized tests are the Test of Written Language (TOWL) (Hammill and Larsen 1978) and the Picture Story Lan-guage Test (PSLT) (Myklebust 1965). Both tests measure aspects of pro-ductivity, such as number of words or sentences, level of vocabulary de-velopment, and ideation, but neither deals with the process of writing. Additional drawbacks that teachers and clinicians should be aware of in administering these tests include the fact that: (1) both tests deal only with the narrative form of written expression; (2) they provide only a one-shot picture of a student's writing ability; and (3) they fail to allow for revision (Bain 1986; Poplin et al. 1980). In addition, both tests suffer from ques-tionable validity and reliability (Poplin et al. 1980).

In diagnosing a student's writing ability we must develop ways to compensate for the inadequacies of the existing standardized tests. Regina Cicci (1983), for example, suggests asking parents and other teachers for samples of a student's writing. For classroom evaluation, we might devise checklists of the component skills of written expression, as both M. J. Weiner (1980) and J. Poteet (1980) have done. Criticizing existing assess-ment devices for placing too much stress on the mechanical skills involved in writing and not enough on "meaningful writing behavior," Mary Pop-lin (1983) urges that writing be viewed from a development perspective, using methods such as primary-trait scoring techniques (Cooper and Odell 1977). In this approach, a writing sample is evaluated holistically and in terms of the degree to which it meets standards for that particular writing task, for example, dialogue, or character description. Poplin has devised an assessment schema of developmental writing activities with suggested assessment measures for each. For younger children, many of these measures are dependent on parent interview, and for older children, teacher observation is frequently required.

HANDWRITING PROBLEMS

Research on handwriting is minimal, and there is no reliable standardized measurement instrument to evaluate letter and word formations (Cicci 1983). Although the TOWL contains a measure of handwriting ability, it is extremely subjective. A diagnostic test of cursive handwriting, The Childrens' Handwriting Evaluation Scale, has recently been developed at Scottish Rite Hospital in Dallas, Texas (Phelps and Stempel 1987) but has not yet been used widely enough to attest to its value. The Zaner-Bloser Company in Columbus, Ohio has developed a set of handwriting evaluation scales for grades one through eight. These scales are meant to be used with the Zaner-Bloser Handwriting Program (1987). Because the scoring criteria are so high, they are really not appropriate for general use.

A significant percentage of dyslexic individuals have poor handwriting; however, the types of problems they exhibit vary in nature and severity. Visual memory deficits, fine motor problems (dysgraphia), or slow rate of execution may all interfere with handwriting (Cicci 1983). It is not far-fetched to suggest that emotional factors may also contribute to poor handwriting, given the lack of confidence most dyslexic people have in their spelling abilities. I often note ambiguous letter formations intended to mask potential spelling errors. Unfortunately, to date no systematic analysis of these difficulties or investigation of their relationship to attending manifestations of dyslexia has been made. Such an investigation might help to determine whether severe handwriting deficits reflect a subtype of dyslexia with neurological involvement, as suggested by Doris Johnson and Helmer Myklebust (1967).

PHONOLOGICAL PROCESSING DEFICITS

Research comparing the phonological abilities of good and poor readers suggests that deficits in phonological processing, which may be more or less subtle, underly the poorer reading and writing skills of dyslexics. Weaknesses in four areas of phonological processing are observed in poor readers (Blachman 1983; Brady and Fowler 1988; Liberman and Shankweiler 1985). These areas include: (1) phonological awareness, or cognizance of the individual sound segments in spoken language; (2) phonetic coding to maintain information in working memory, which can be conceptualized as short-term verbal memory; (3) phonetic perception to create a phonological code, otherwise referred to as auditory perception of speech sounds; and (4) phonological recoding in lexical access, or the ability to retrieve names for symbolic stimuli. According to Brady and

Fowler, there are strong correlations between weaknesses in any one of these phonological abilities at kindergarten level and later reading disability.

Deficits in Phonological Awareness.   We have considerable evidence that dyslexic readers are less aware than good readers of the discrete phonological elements within words and thereby less able to segment words into their component parts. In Chapter 1, I indicated that linguistic segmentation ability develops from larger to smaller units, from words within sentences, to syllables within words, and finally phonemes within syllables (see page 8). It is this last, finer discrimination that appears to be the stumbling block for dyslexic readers. Isabelle Liberman and her colleagues (1977), Barbara Fox and Donald Routh (1980; 1983) and other investigative teams have shown that children in the early grades who are delayed in acquiring phonemic analysis skills (segmenting and blending) are poor readers at follow-up several years later. Susan Brady and Anne Fowler (1988) call attention to the fact that the ability to "reflect on the structure of words" and to segment and blend phonemes requires conscious awareness (also referred to as metalinguistic awareness), whereas other phonological processes involved in reading and writing occur at a subconscious level. As I mentioned in Chapter 1, one of the most provocative questions in reading research today is whether phonological awareness develops independently of reading or whether it develops as a result of experience with print. The answer to this question has crucial implications for the prevention of reading failure.

Short-Term Verbal Memory Deficits.   There is abundant evidence that dyslexic readers have difficulty processing verbal information in memory; the problem seems not to apply to nonverbal information, such as memory for faces (Liberman et al. 1980; Nelson and Warrington 1980). Memory differences between dyslexic and normally achieving readers appear only with stimuli that must be linguistically coded (Mann 1986).

The greatest memory differences between very poor and proficient readers show up on tasks that involve retention of verbal information in short-term memory (also called working memory), particularly for serial order recall of lists of items such as digits, letters, words, and objects or pictures that must be named (Blachman 1983; Lorsbach and Gray 1985; Moore et al. 1982). It is now widely believed that units of verbal information are held in short-term memory in phonological form while that information, be it lists or sentences, is being processed (see page 21). Isabelle Liberman and her colleagues have conducted numerous studies that suggest disabled readers do not utilize the phonological code to hold letters and words in short-term memory (Liberman, et al. 1977). They are less able than good readers to remember strings of unrelated letters or words as flashed on a screen by a tachistoscope. Additionally, their performance does not decline, like that of good readers, when these strings include phonetically confusable items, as for example, *B, C, D,* which Liberman and her associates interpret as another indication of their failure to store verbal information phonologically. This weakness may be directly related not only to decoding problems but also to the comprehension problems evidenced by dyslexic readers (Brady and Fowler 1988).

Although we have ample proof that verbal memory deficits contribute to reading disabilities, we are faced with another chicken and egg question. Are phonological encoding deficits the source of processing problems in short-term memory or do problems of primary processing in short-term memory impinge on acquisition of the phonemic code?

Speech Perception Deficits. The suggestion that the problems dyslexic people have with phonological processing may lie at the level of perception, as well as conceptualization (Brady and Fowler 1988), derives some, though not extensive, support from the research. Dyslexic children have demonstrated inferior auditory perception of speech sounds relative to normal children but only under distractible conditions, where the stimulus was presented against background noise (Brady, Shankweiler, and Mann 1983). No differences have been found between dyslexic and nondyslexic children in perception of nonverbal environmental sounds (Brady, Shankweiler, and Mann 1983; Godfrey et al. 1981) which tends to rule out the possibility that dyslexics have a generalized auditory impairment.

Paula Tallal (1980), however, who is noted for her work with language impaired children, observed a group of reading impaired children, not diagnosed as language impaired, who were deficient in discriminating tone sequences presented at rapid rates. Tallal and her colleague, Rachel Stark, (Tallal and Stark 1982) suggest that there may be a subgroup of dyslexic individuals having a subtle auditory perceptual deficit characterized by difficulty in perceiving and analyzing rapidly presented speech sounds. They believe that this problem would interfere with the ability to detect the finer discriminations between phonemes in words and consequently with the ability to make connections between graphemes and phonemes in attempting to read.

Before we can draw any meaningful conclusions about speech perception deficits in dyslexic individuals, we need to know the prevalence of such problems among this group of disabled readers, as well as more about the severity of the deficits and the extent to which they affect learning in areas other than reading. Furthermore, we need to know if disabled readers who manifest these deficiencies suffer from a specific subtype of dyslexia or whether they are simply more seriously affected by the disorder.

Name Retrieval Deficits. Dyslexic people are slower at naming series of various types of familiar stimulus items—objects, colors, numbers, and letters. This task, first developed as a test by Martha Denckla and Rita Rudel (1976a, 1976b), distinguishes dyslexic subjects from other learning disabled subjects, as well as from normally achieving subjects.

Somewhat earlier, Jeannette Jansky and Katrina de Hirsch (1972) determined that children with severe reading problems have difficulty naming
single familiar picture items. Denckla and Rudel (1976b) support this finding by showing that dyslexic children make more errors in naming line
drawings than normal or nondyslexic learning disabled children. Most of
their errors are circumlocutions, rather than omissions or misnomers, indicating that they know something about the pictured object but cannot
produce the name. The proposed explanation for these naming difficulties
is that dyslexic people have trouble accessing the phonological representation of words in the lexicon. This hypothesized process has been referred
to as *phonological recoding in lexical access* (Brady and Fowler 1988; Wagner
and Torgesen 1987).

Continuous naming tasks, such as Denckla and Rudel's Rapid Automatic Naming (RAN) test, tend to be more sensitive to ability differences than single-item naming tasks (Stanovich 1985); yet both types of
tasks have been incorporated into screening batteries for identifying dyslexic children (Blachman 1983, 1984; German 1984; Jansky and de Hirsch
1972; Wolf 1984). We must use discretion in the application and interpretation of naming tasks for diagnosing dyslexia, as questions still need to be
answered concerning the processes and deficits involved in these naming
tasks, particularly in the continuous type task. As Charles Perfetti (1985a)
observed, it is not yet clear whether the problem for dyslexic individuals
lies in the speed of word retrieval or in rapid sequential naming, nor is it
apparent to what extent visual scanning, articulatory mechanisms, or
memory factors are implicated in the breakdown.

DYSLEXIA AND EARLY LANGUAGE DEFICITS

Research substantiates a significant relationship between early language processing and/or production problems severe enough to be diagnosed as such and later reading disabilities. Follow-up studies of children
diagnosed as having specific language impairment (SLI) have shown the
incidence of later reading disability to be 90 percent or greater (Stark et al.
1984; Strominger and Bashir 1977). However, most dyslexics do not demonstrate these overt language impairments. At the same time, as Paula
Menyuk and James Flood (1981) observe, most of them do exhibit less dis-
cernible language-based deficits, such as phonological processing problems and lack of metalinguistic awareness described above.

VISUAL PROBLEMS AND DYSLEXIA
THE VISUAL-PERCEPTUAL DEFICIT HYPOTHESIS

Unfortunately, the stereotyped impression of a dyslexic person as
someone who reads and writes letters backward and/or upside down,

which is often referred to as mirror reading, continues. True, some dyslexic individuals do demonstrate this unique behavior; as I previously mentioned, word reading errors such as word and letter substitutions, letter reversals, and letter sequencing confusions are common among dyslexic people. Given that these types of errors are the most overt sign of reading problems, it is not surprising that dyslexia was first construed as a problem rooted in the visual system. James Hinshelwood (1917), for example, refers to the problem as *"congenital word blindness."* Samuel Orton (1925; 1937), a neurologist, calls the problem "strephosymbolia," or *twisted symbols.* He attributes the problem to incomplete cerebral dominance and the failure of one hemisphere of the brain to suppress the mirror images of the letter symbols transferred from the other. Orton maintains that in all individuals mirror images are received by the nondominant hemisphere, but that in normal readers the dominant hemisphere takes over in processing visual stimuli.

Orton's theory of mirror image repression has since been discredited on several grounds, one being that reversal and sequencing errors do not account for a greater proportion of the total reading errors made by dyslexic readers than by normal readers (Stanovich 1986a). Another reason to question the visual perceptual deficit hypothesis is that disabled readers do not differ from normal readers in their performance on nonlinguistic tasks, such as the ability to distinguish visual designs or faces (Liberman and Shankweiler 1979). In studies performed by Frank Vellutino and his colleagues (Vellutino 1983; Vellutino et al. 1975; Vellutino, Steger, and Kandel 1972), poor readers had no more difficulty than good readers in copying or recognizing letters or words from a novel alphabet, which were essentially nonverbal stimuli. Furthermore, Vellutino (1978, 1983) has demonstrated that poor readers are almost as adept as good readers at copying visually confusable letters and words from memory, although they are significantly inferior at naming or pronouncing these items on second exposure. He attributes their naming problems to less well established verbal codes for letter or word forms rather than to visual perception deficits. Vellutino (1987) suggests that the mirror writing exhibited by some dyslexics (as well as some normally developing readers) reflects their incomplete grasp of letter-sound relationships rather than a visuo-spatial disorder. He feels that this weakness precludes the positive writing experiences that normally foster knowledge of directional and positional cues in letters.

There are two more reasons to reject the visual perceptual deficit explanation for dyslexia. The first is that visual perceptual training is generally ineffective in improving the reading skills of dyslexic individuals (Bateman 1979; Bryant 1979). The second is that no significant correlation has been established between early visuo-spatial or visuo-motor problems and later reading ability (Robinson and Schwartz 1973).

OCULAR FUSION PROBLEMS

Because erratic eye movement patterns have been observed in disabled readers, it has been hypothesized that dyslexia is caused by unstable ocular dominance (Pavlidis 1985; Punnet and Steinhauer 1984). However, it seems more likely that erratic eye movement is the result, rather than the cause of reading problems, because in most cases it is not observed when poor readers are reading at their independent reading levels. At the same time, researchers who have made these observations feel that there may be a small percentage of dyslexic readers whose abnormal fixation patterns reflect a primary visual–spatial disorder (Benton 1985; Keogh and Pelland 1985; Raynor 1985).

Optometric training programs that proliferated in the 1960s have been generally unsuccessful in promoting reading acquisition (Keogh and Pelland 1985; Metzger and Werner 1984), although some researchers attest to their positive effects with qualifications. For example, A. F. Punnet and G. D. Steinhauer (1984) claim that ocular training improved the reading comprehension of their four experimental subjects, but only when training was combined with verbal reinforcement.

We have by no means resolved all questions regarding the implication of visual problems in dyslexia; two of particular importance need to be answered. The first is whether there is a small subtype of dyslexia represented by a fundamental visuo–spatial disorder, as suggested by Arthur Benton (1985), Charles Perfetti (1985b), and others. The second is whether the reading difficulties of this hypothetical subtype are direct consequences of dyslexia or concurrent manifestations of a more central neurological dysfunction.

THE INTERSENSORY DEFICIT HYPOTHESIS

Another hypothesized explanation for dyslexia is that dyslexic individuals have a problem integrating information that must be processed simultaneously in two or more modalities (Birch 1962). This makes sense, for in reading, both auditory and visual systems are involved.

Herbert Birch, who first proposed the intersensory deficit hypothesis, developed a test of auditory-visual integration that requires children to match rhythmic patterns with dot patterns, and found that some poor readers were markedly less proficient than good readers at this task (Birch and Belmont 1964). However, subsequent efforts by Birch and his associates to substantiate this theory have been criticized for failing to control for deficiencies within, rather than between, sensory channels (Bryant 1968). Other researchers, such as Naomi Zigmond (1966), find that disabled readers are inferior to normal readers when processing information in a single modality, as on auditory tasks; therefore, their inferior performance on intersensory tasks can be expected.

In a further challenge to the intersensory or cross modal deficit hypothesis, Frank Vellutino and his colleagues (Vellutino, Steger, and Pruzek 1973) find no significant differences between poor and normal readers on nonverbal paired-associate matching tasks which measure both within and between modality functioning (visual-visual; auditory-auditory, visual-auditory), whereas, similar studies carried out with verbal stimuli, such as words and letters, reveal notable differences for reader type. These investigators conclude that verbal, rather than intersensory, deficits distinguish dyslexics from normal readers.

Despite the research findings that appear to rule out the implication of intersensory deficits in dyslexia, the jury is still out on this issue. In the last decade, neurologists and psychologists have been investigating the possibility of neuronal pathway disconnections in the brain as a possible cause of dyslexia. These disconnections may manifest themselves in more subtle ways than previously imagined and therefore may not be sensitive to experiments such as those cited above (Denckla 1987).

SUBTYPES OR UNITARY DISORDER?

Because the symptoms ascribed to dyslexia range in severity and are not apparent in all individuals presumed to be dyslexic, the syndrome appears to be a heterogenous disorder. A question that has provoked specialists and researchers for some time is whether dyslexia is a unique syndrome or whether it comprises a number of identifiable subcategories. The question has led to studies aimed at classifying dyslexia into discrete subtypes based on patterns of symptoms.

Subtyping research began more than twenty years ago with M. Kinsbourne and E. K. Warrington. They distinguish two groups of disabled readers having more than a twenty point discrepancy between verbal and performance IQ on the Wechsler Intelligence Scale (Duane 1983a): Children with lower verbal IQs appear to have language related deficits, whereas those with lower performance IQs demonstrate perceptual and visual-motor impairments. As previously mentioned (pages 23–24), Elena Boder (1971), as well as Rebecca Treiman and Jonathan Baron (1983), categorize disabled readers according to spelling strategies, Boder distinguishing dysphonetic and dyseidetic subtypes, and Treiman and Baron making a similar distinction which they refer to as Phoenecian and Chinese. In the last eight years there has been a proliferation of classification studies using more advanced statistical techniques such as Q-factor analysis and cluster analysis. However, the results of these studies overall are more confounding than enlightening. For example, in specifying six categories, Rymantas Petrauskas and Byron Rourke (1979) acknowledge one to be "unreliable" (13 percent of subjects) and another to comprise subjects who are unclassifiable (32 percent).

Most of the early classification studies, such as Boder's, focused on the search for a single shared deficit among dyslexic subgroups (Lovett 1984). The more recent multifactorial studies fall into two categories: those that examine reading behaviors and those that, having a psycho-neurological perspective, test other cognitive, nonreading skills. In both cases, investigators look for performance patterns "which may suggest different problems associated with and presumed to cause the child's reading disability" (Lovett 1984). The result is often that a significant number of cases do not fall into any distinct patterns or clusters, as Petrauskas and Rourke (1979) found.

Limitations noted in the subtyping research conducted thus far include the use of psychometrically weak tests (Doehring 1984) and the absence of control groups (Lundberg 1985). The most serious failing of classification investigations is the lack of information they have provided on how the identified processing deficits affect the reading process itself (Lovett 1984). After conducting a number of subtyping studies, Donald Doehring declared himself disenchanted with subtyping methodology that uses group comparisons. A more productive approach, in his view, would involve individual case studies (Doehring 1984).

Charles Perfetti (1985b) has taken another position on the issue of ability differences among reading disabled individuals. He suggests that dyslexia may represent a point at the extreme low end of a continuum of reading disability rather than a unique disorder with specific causality. A follow-up study in England on adults who had experienced early reading problems lends support to this thesis (Scarborough 1984). The study found few consistent qualitative differences to distinguish those predetermined to be dyslexic, based on IQ-reading discrepancy data, and those considered to be poor readers. H. S. Scarborough, the author of the study, concluded that the relation of dyslexia to other reading problems may be a matter of degree rather than kind. Other respected reading researchers holding this point of view include Richard Olson (Olson et al. 1985) and Keith Stanovich (1986a).

Despite the imprecise and ambivalent outcome of most of the dyslexia classification studies, there are two significant findings. The first is that in the majority of these studies language related deficits stand out as the most prevalent characteristic of dyslexia (Boder 1971; Denckla 1977; Mattis, French, and Rapin 1975; Olson et al. 1985; Petraukas and Rourke 1979; Satz and Morris 1980; Treiman and Baron 1983). Acknowledging this overall finding, Perfetti (1985) has proposed that the continuum of reading ability is based on the level of acquisition and application of the phonetic code in conjunction with linguistic memory. The second significant finding is that in most of these classification studies a distinct subtype best characterized as a *visual-spatial type* has appeared. Although this subtype accounted for a relatively small portion of the deficit categories, it must nevertheless be recognized.

Without doubt the diversity in dyslexia symptomology deserves further exploration; answers to our questions on this subject have direct bearing on the identification and treatment of dyslexia. The Orton Dyslexia Society, the leading national organization concerned with dyslexia, recently endorsed the concept that there is not one but many dyslexias (Leong and Enfield 1986).

NEUROLOGICAL FACTORS IN DYSLEXIA

Overt neurological problems are not usually present among dyslexic children (Rutter 1978). Therefore, investigative efforts to understand the neurological underpinnings of dyslexia have focused primarily on behavioral differences in individuals, thought to indicate divergences in hemispheric specialization. The basic assumption behind this research is that language processing in dyslexics may not be controlled by the same areas of the brain as in nondyslexic individuals. For the majority of the population, these areas lie in the left cerebral hemisphere. Much of this research has examined *laterality differences* presumed to reflect *lateralization differences*. By "laterality" we mean the choice of hand, eye, or foot in performing everyday activities, more precisely defined as "the voluntary use of the peripheral nervous system in executing some motor, spatial, or verbal function" (Obrzut and Boliek 1986). "Lateralization" refers to "the involuntary brain functioning of the left and/or right cerebral hemispheres" (Obrzut and Boliek 1986), otherwise called hemispheric specialization.

LATERALITY DIFFERENCES

The relationship between left-handedness and reading disbility has received considerable attention; however, the overall findings related to this issue are extremely inconsistent. Much of the problem is due to the fact that handedness is not easily measured but rather appears to rest on a continuum ranging from strong right-handedness to mixed-handedness to strong left-handedness (Hardyck and Petrinovich 1977). Furthermore, hand preference can be affected by familial, cultural, or educational influences. Because it deviates from the norm, left-handedness is more susceptible to these influences and thus less reliably identified than right-handedness.

Within the general population, the incidence of left-handedness has been estimated to be 8 to 10 percent (Kinsbourne and Hiscock 1981); lateralization indices are not as easily determined. Drake Duane, a neurologist, reported in 1983 that 98 percent of right-handed people and 70 percent of left-handed people have language lateralized in the left hemisphere (Duane 1983b). An interesting finding from one study (Hardyck and Petronovich 1977) is that left-handers with a family history of left-handedness appear to have less hemispheric specialization than right-handers, whereas left-handers with no family history of left-handedness seem to process language in the left hemisphere like most right-handers. Confounding the issue is the possibility that some cases of left-handedness may be the result of early brain injury (Satz, Saslow, and Henry 1985). Clinical investigations of reading disorder may involve such "pathological left-handers" and cognitive deficits in such cases would more likely be due to cerebral insult than to deviant cerebral lateralization (Hiscock and Kinsbourne 1982). Any data pertaining to the connection between left-handedness and dyslexia, therefore, would be falsely skewed.

Among educators, psychologists, and neuropsychologists opinions on the theorized association between handedness patterns and reading disability vary considerably. Finding left-handedness to be more common in males than females, the late Norman Geschwind, a neurologist who pioneered neurological research on the etiology of dyslexia, proposed a theory based on epidemiological research, which links male sex, left-handedness, and autoimmune diseases to dyslexia (Geschwind and Behan 1982). Further exploration of this hypothesized association is being carried out by Geschwind's colleagues at Beth Israel Hospital in Boston, principally Albert Galaburda (Galaburda 1985). The majority opinion among respected professionals exploring the link between left-handedness and dyslexia, however, is that we lack enough substantial data to draw definitive conclusions (Hiscock and Kinsbourne 1982).

In contrast to the unresolved issues related to handedness and dyslexia, the research indicates quite firmly that there is no significant link between eye preference and reading disability (Hiscock and Kinsbourne 1982; Obrzut and Boliek 1986; Rutter 1978). The prevalence of cross eye-hand functioning in the normal population is approximately 30 percent (Kinsbourne and Hiscock 1981). Footedness is more strongly related to handedness but is not a reliable predictor of reading achievement or of cognitive functioning (Hiscock and Kinsbourne 1982; Rutter 1978).

LATERALIZATION DIFFERENCES

Several measures of central language processing have been devised that are now considered to be better indices of cerebral lateralization than handedness. One of these measures is dichotic listening, where paired stimuli are presented simultaneously to each ear and the subject's response pattern, favoring one or the other ear, is thought to indicate the dominant hemisphere for that particular stimulus type: a right-ear advantage (REA) reflecting left-hemispheric processing and vice versa. Another measure, visual half-field (VHF) technique, involves presenting verbal or nonverbal stimuli tachistoscopically to either the left or right visual fields, or to both fields simultaneously in bilateral presentations. Response performance comparisons are considered to reflect degree of lateralization to one or the other hemisphere. A third procedure, verbal-manual time-sharing technique, compares simultaneous performance on tasks presumed to involve the same hemisphere (e.g., speaking and a manual activity performed with the right hand) and tasks involving separate hemispheres (e.g., speaking and left hand activities). Normal individuals exhibit diminished performance under both conditions, but to a greater degree when activities are directed toward the same as opposed to separate hemispheres. The theory behind the use of any of these techniques is that differences in response patterns will distinguish dyslexics from nondyslexics. Unfortunately, none of these methods has yielded consistent results, due in some part to methodological problems (Obrzut and Boliek 1986).

Although we do not have reliable evidence of language lateralization differences in dyslexics, several technological advances have considerable potential in this regard. One is the development of event-related potential (ERP) methods, which record electrical activity as the subject performs specific tasks (Shucard et al. 1985). Brain electrical activity mapping (BEAM) is another promising technique (Denckla 1986; Duffy et al. 1980).

CEREBRAL ANOMALIES

Efforts to look still more directly for possible cerebral abnormalities in dyslexic individuals have involved a number of noninvasive techniques, such as electroencephalography (EEG), an electrical scanning procedure, and computerized tomography (CT), a radiological scanning technique. So far, neither of these brain scanning methods has been effective in identifying dyslexia (Connors 1978, Denckla 1978; Denckla, LeMay, and Chapman 1985; Duane 1983b).

A few postmortem anatomical studies have been conducted on the brains of persons previously diagnosed as dyslexic (Galaburda 1983, 1985; Galaburda and Kemper 1979). Although biological anomalies were indicated, the number of cases (five to date) are not enough to draw any definitive conclusions about the occurrence of cerebral abnormalities in dyslexics (Geschwind 1986). However, in the opinion of the investigators, one finding is considered particularly significant: Whereas in most individuals the left hemisphere is larger than the right, in the four dyslexic brains examined for this dimension, "all four showed deviation from the standard assymmetry pattern of the language regions, i.e., instead of a larger size of the left temporal language region there was symmetry" (Galaburda 1985). The symmetry appears due to a larger than normal right hemisphere in the dyslexic brains. This finding has led Albert Galaburda to postulate that the etiology of dyslexia lies in abnormal migration of neural cells during fetal development.

WHAT WE KNOW AND DON'T KNOW ABOUT DYSLEXIA

We know that dyslexia is a disability pertaining to the processing of written language. This includes both reading and writing. Although dyslexia is often perceived as a visual problem, overwhelming evidence indicates that it is a language based disorder; deficiencies in the ability to process the phonology of our language seem to lie at its core. These deficiencies are not correlated with IQ—dyslexics can fall at any point on the intelligence curve, and many, in fact, place at the superior end.

Dyslexic readers do not readily acquire metalinguistic knowledge; they are less aware of the units of sound in spoken language than good readers and less able to conceptualize the translation of those sound units into written symbols and vice versa. Thus they have trouble grasping the phonetically based alphabetic code and mastering the letter-sound correspondences of the English alphabet. This problem interferes most with their ability to decode unfamiliar words. Despite the fact that dyslexic readers usually learn to identify a number of words on sight, their word recognition is slower and less accurate than that of able readers. To the extent that decoding problems limit their reading speed and accuracy, as well as their ability to utilize the surrounding context to facilitate word recognition, the reading comprehension of dyslexic individuals is jeopardized. Persons with dyslexia have at least as much difficulty encoding as decoding words; poor spelling is one of the most persistent indicators of dyslexia and by far the most prevalent of their problems with written expression. Whereas all dyslexic people suffer from the deficiencies cited above, they do so in varying degrees. Their symptoms may be more or less evident, depending upon the severity of the deficiencies, as well as on the presence or absence of compensating abilities. Most dyslexic people exhibit poor short-term memory for verbal information. Based on research evidence, it appears that this weakness is attributable to their phonological processing deficits. It also appears that poor short-term verbal memory, rather than cognitive deficits, may account for the problems some dyslexics have with written language syntax.

Overt language impairment does not usually accompany dyslexia; however, many dyslexic individuals evidence name retrieval problems and some have demonstrated subtle speech perception deficits. Furthermore, children diagnosed as language impaired are almost certain to have later reading disabilities.

Dyslexic children and adults do tend to reverse and transpose letters and words, but in no greater proportion to their overall reading and writing errors than nondyslexic people. Earlier construed as evidence of a visual perceptual disorder, such errors in most cases of dyslexia can be explained by unstable letter-sound knowledge. At the same time, a small percentage of dyslexic individuals do appear to have specific visual-spatial deficits, and some, but by no means all, manifest grapho-motor problems.

At the present time, we do not know whether the variations observed among the manifestations of dyslexia represent differences in degree or type of disability. The question remains, are there one or many dyslexias? The answer is critical for remedial, as well as for identification purposes.

Dyslexia is a neurologically based disorder in which language areas of the brain must be implicated. We do not know the precise locations of the dysfunction within these areas, nor what other brain mechanisms are involved and how. Such information, when it is acquired, should go a long way toward understanding the etiology of dyslexia. In the meantime, we need to devote at least as much attention to mitigating the effects of dyslexia as to determining its cause.

PART

Remedial Instruction

CHAPTER

Principles and Techniques of Remedial Instruction for Dyslexic Students

Although we should not minimize the importance of understanding the nature of dyslexia, reading disabilities research has been justifiably criticized for focusing disproportionately on the search for causality and all but neglecting inquiry on correction or prevention of the problem (Bryant et al. 1980; Chall 1978; Lipson and Wixson 1986). The reading disabilities field has in fact been referred to as "deficit driven" (Poplin 1983). Rachel Gittelman, a psychologist at College of Physicians and Surgeons, Columbia University, reviewing the research on the remediation of reading disorders, states "The literature on the treatment of children with reading retardation is full of opinionated practices devoid of even barely adequately controlled treatment research." (Gittelman 1983).

There are several plausible explanations for the relative lack of treatment research on dyslexia, the first being the effort and cost involved; the need for a remedy is usually urgent, therefore taking precedence over the need to plan for later evaluation. A second explanation is that many remedial programs began in the private sector where formal evaluation is not required for implementation, as it is in many public school systems. Still another reason is that few of the more popular programs or techniques have been affiliated with a college or university where research is routinely conducted. Moreover, much of the research that does exist is methodologically flawed, as a task force of the Research Institute for the Study of Learning Disabilities at Columbia University Teachers College

43

discovered in surveying the research literature (Peister et al. 1978–1980). Gittelman points out that small numbers of subjects in the sample populations, lack of control groups, and failure to randomly assign subjects to treatment and control groups, are some of the design problems in the studies to date (Gittelman 1983).

Random assignment to treatment groups is particularly difficult to achieve, since dyslexic subjects are often already in treatment. The length of time needed to produce significant gains from remedial instruction, which is usually two years or more (Peister et al. 1978–1980), also tends to discourage practitioners from carrying out effectiveness studies. Furthermore, in many studies, as Gittelman notes, neither the duration nor the intensity of treatment is spelled out, calling into question any conclusions that may be drawn.

The Teachers College task force (Peister et al. 1978–1980) has drawn attention to the fact that even where control or comparison groups exist, the instruction applied in these groups is often not adequately described, making it difficult to determine which instructional components are actually being compared. The nature of choice of outcome measures frequently is not given adequate consideration in planning program evaluation or in interpreting findings from studies that have been carried out. As Gittelman (1983) points out, most standardized tests are not designed to pick up small gains over short periods of time; thus, with short term or "one shot" studies the possibility of failure to detect treatment effects statistically where they exist is greatly increased. I will be mentioning these and other methodological problems as I discuss studies on remedial instruction for dyslexics.

As teachers and instructional decision makers for dyslexic children, it is important that we try to ascertain the effectiveness of any remedial method or technique before initiating or advocating its use. This is not always possible, as I have indicated. However, where treatment evaluation studies have been done, we need to keep in mind the potential methodological problems that I have discussed and exert caution in interpreting the results.

DIRECT INSTRUCTION

Despite the lack of empirical support, there is remarkable consensus on the major principles to be applied in remedial treatment for dyslexic students (Bryant et al. 1980). One of the most acknowledged principles is direct instruction. N. G. Haring and B. Bateman in their book, *Teaching the Learning Disabled Child* (1977), make the point that dyslexic children do not learn "by osmosis," as other children seem to do. Rather, they need direct, intensive, and systematic input from, and interaction with, the teacher.

Three different models of direct instruction have been applied to dyslexic children: the tutoring model (Traub 1982), the small group model (Cox 1985; Enfield and Greene 1981), and the whole class model (Wolf 1985). Determining which of these models is most effective and most economically efficient is one of the critical challenges facing us in the field of reading disabilities.

Nancy Karweit of Johns Hopkins University suggests that we judge the relative value of the different models of adaptive instruction in terms of *student use of instructional time* (Karweit 1985). This concept has been referred to alternatively as academic learning time (Berliner 1981), academic engaged time (Ysseldyke and Algozzine 1983), and time on task (Otto, Wolf, and Eldridge 1984). In reviewing the drawbacks and advantages of different educational settings, Karweit adopts J. B. Carroll's definition of learning time as the ratio of time spent to time needed (when the two factors are equivalent, learning is maximized) (Carroll 1963). In the whole-class model, Karweit notes that the amount of active learning time varies widely with the size and heterogeneity of the class and the procedural demands on the teacher. However, in this model all teaching time can be devoted to direct instruction.

In the within-class grouping approach, instructional time for each group is divided between direct instruction and independent seat work. While reducing the amount of direct instruction for each student, this approach can place an excessive burden on teachers, because they must monitor seat work in addition to working directly with each group. Looking at individualized instruction only within a classroom setting (a model, she notes, that is considerably less popular today), Karweit emphasizes the formidable management problems involved in distributing teacher time and the often large amount of time wasted in students' waiting for the teacher's attention. Although she does not attempt to confirm the superiority of one instructional model over another, Karweit provides an important perspective on classroom management.

Dyslexic students need more time to learn than nondisabled students (Haring and Bateman 1977), and special educators have given considerable thought to the issue of academic engaged time. For example, Wayne Otto and his colleagues (1984) have concluded that this variable is the best predictor of academic achievement; James Ysseldyke and Bob Algozzine (1983) suggest that reading diagnosis should begin with an examination of student time on task. Ethna Reid (1986), in designing an instructional program to be used in classrooms to prevent reading failure, makes provisions for minimizing the length of teacher questions and student response latencies in order to maximize learning time. Unison oral response is incorporated in several programs (for example, Distar and Slingerland) to ensure that each student is fully involved in the lesson at hand. The use of teacher scripts (Calfee 1981–1984; Engelmann and Bruner 1983; Reid

1986) can be viewed as another approach to time management. These scripts are written formats provided to teachers to help structure their lessons. Scripts may be more or less specific; in the DISTAR program (see Chapter 17), for example, the scripts tell teachers exactly what to say and do during each lesson, when to call for responses, when to repeat statements for emphasis or correction, and so on, thereby controlling the pace of instruction.

Careful pacing of instruction is an essential feature of effective teaching for dyslexic students in order to prevent information overload, which occurs "when the amount of information to be processed within a given time span exceeds the individual's capacity" (Bryant et al. 1980). N. D. Bryant and his associates (1980) have identified four processing problems that contribute to overloading: (1) slow speed of processing, (2) difficulty automatizing information learned, (3) failure to apply strategies, and (4) distractibility. The successful teacher or practitioner working with dyslexic students, regardless of instructional setting, must provide for this contingency in planning each lesson (Cox 1984; Gillingham and Stillman 1960; Slingerland 1976). Most established remedial methods and programs utilize a structured, hierarchical approach to learning, breaking down tasks into small units taught in order of difficulty (Bryant et al. 1980).

LEARNING TO MASTERY

Mastery is an extremely important factor in remedial or preventive instruction for disabled learners. Barak Rosenshine, who supports direct teaching, states that, to ensure retention, mastery needs to reach levels of 70 to 80 percent when new reading skills are acquired; in independent practice, mastery should be 100 percent, especially for disabled learners (Rosenshine 1983). David Berliner, another strong advocate of direct instruction, maintains that younger and less able students need to achieve almost errorless performance on early learning tasks in order for later learning to be successful (Berliner 1981).

Gaining automaticity is a critical component of mastery learning in remedial reading instruction. Automatic processing at the word level frees up working memory to allow for more efficient processing at the sentence and passage levels of text (LaBerge and Samuels 1974; Perfetti 1985a; Stanovich 1984). As mentioned earlier, dyslexic readers in general are markedly slower at word recognition than good readers (Perfetti 1984; Stanovich 1980). Most of the established remedial programs for dyslexic students, therefore, make ample provision for extended practice to attain automaticity beginning at the letter-sound level. Barbara Bateman in particular stresses the need for repetition with all new learning, a concept termed "overlearning" (Bateman 1979). However, as N. D. Bryant and his associates at Teachers College point out, practice needs to be carefully distributed over time, rather than massed. They suggest that "massed practice reinforces short-term memory at the expense of long-term memory" (Bryant et al. 1980). The majority of remedial programs for dyslexic students provide for systematic review of previously learned material at the beginning and end of each lesson.

Prompting techniques are often utilized in treatment approaches to decrease the possibility of errors and to help students to respond without overcontrolling their behavior (DeCecco 1968). Although there has not been much research of the subject, Bryant and his associates (1980) report on two studies that support the value of prompting in remedial instruction which usually involves using picture or object cues as memory aids. For example, remedial programs derived from the Orton-Gillingham approach (see Chapters 12 and 14) provide pictures to promote letter-sound associations (a picture of a pig for the letter *p*, for instance).

Academic feedback is another essential instructional component of learning to mastery (Berliner 1981). B. Rosenshine and R. Stevens (1984) cite immediate feedback from the teacher as one of the five most important contributive factors to academic achievement. They subdivide the feedback process into four instructional components: demonstration, guided practice, feedback, and independent practice. Although little research has specifically investigated the effects of this variable on dyslexic students, some provision for feedback is incorporated in all established programs. It is not necessarily teacher driven, however, as in the classic Direct Instruction model exemplified by the DISTAR program (Engelmann and Bruner 1983) (see Chapter 17). In some programs, a discovery, or Socratic, method is used (Cox 1984; Lindamood and Lindamood 1975), albeit under careful teacher supervision to ensure correct responses. When working with older students, frequent performance assessment offers a way to inform them of their progress, thereby increasing motivation (Zigmond and Miller 1986). Providing standards against which to measure their performance also helps students to become self-monitors and take on more responsibility for their own progress (Bandura 1982).

Gaining pupil attention is particularly important in teaching dyslexic children who are prone to distraction (Bryant et al. 1980) and often lack motivation due to previous failure (King 1985). Techniques to promote attending behavior have been incorporated into many instructional programs for these students. For example, the Alphabetic Phonics and Slingerland programs (see Chapters 12 and 14) require specific sitting positions to be assumed before reading and writing activities begin. Hand signals used to cue group response, as in the DISTAR program and Enfield and Greene's Project Read (see Chapter 16), also serve as attentional devices.

Monitoring and evaluating student progress is an essential component of successful academic treatment, although not all treatment methods for dyslexic students include evaluation procedures. Naomi Zigmond and Sandra Miller (1986) report on studies that showed significantly greater academic gains for students whose teachers monitored student progress, as compared to students whose teachers collected no ongoing progress data. However, these reviewers emphasize that to be effective, progress evaluation must be frequent and systematic and teachers must use the data constructively to modify instruction when needed. Furthermore, a data based approach has been found to be more effective in improving pupil achievement than informal observational procedures, though the data analysis need not be elaborate to provide adequate information on student progress.

MULTISENSORY TECHNIQUES

The use of multisensory techniques in remedial intervention with dyslexic children is widespread and dates back to the 1920s with Grace Fernald who had reading impaired students trace letters or words while saying the names aloud (Fernald and Keller 1921). This procedure came to be known as the VAKT approach (visual, auditory, kinesthetic, tactile). Fernald maintained that VAKT reinforcement would help to produce a memory schema for the stimulus information. Samuel Orton's hypothesis that dyslexia is caused by incomplete cerebral dominance, resulting in reversal and sequencing problems, led to the adoption of multisensory teaching methods by his many disciples (Cox 1984; Gillingham and Stillman 1960; Slingerland 1971; Traub and Bloom 1975). The prototype of multisensory instruction for dyslexic children was developed by Orton's colleague, Anna Gillingham, a psychologist, and is most often referred to as the Orton-Gillingham approach. Gillingham collaborated with Bessie Stillman, a remedial reading teacher, in writing a manual that describes this method (Gillingham and Stillman 1960).

Among these practitioners, the assumed rationale for multisensory remedial training has been that kinesthetic activities help to establish visual-auditory associations in grapheme-phoneme correspondence learning, as well as to reinforce left-to-right letter progression (Orton 1966). Aylett Cox, author of Alphabetic Phonics (see Chapter 12), a program derived from the Orton-Gillingham approach, refers to this learning procedure as "intersensory elaboration." Other proposed benefits of VAKT or VAK techniques are that they encourage attention to details within letters or words (Gates 1927) and that they help in retrieving words from long-term memory (Slingerland 1971).

As the Teachers College task force (Peister et al. 1980) has observed, there were considerable differences in specific techniques among the earlier practitioners of multisensory training. Orton, for example, stated that individual phonic sounds should be pronounced as the child traced a word; Gillingham believed that letter names should be called out; Fernald maintained that words should not be broken up artificially, and that whole words should be said aloud while tracing or writing. Today there is general agreeement among practitioners of Orton-Gillingham derived methods that letter sounds are pronounced when reading words and letter names when spelling (Cox 1984; Enfield 1976). However, even among these programs there are variations in the degree of multisensory input incorporated in teaching procedures. Cox (1985), for example, in order to emphasize precise speech sounds, uses mirrors to demonstrate different oral positions in pronouncing these sounds. Charles and Pat Lindamood (Lindamood and Lindamood 1975) stress the importance of developing oral-motor awareness in children and adults with deficits in auditory conceptualization.

Despite the widespread inclusion of multisensory techniques in remedial programs for dyslexic students and the almost unanimous conviction among practitioners using these techniques that they work, we have little empirical data to validate their effectiveness. We have substantial evidence that many of the programs incorporating these techniques are effective, but we cannot be sure that it is the multisensory factor that makes the significant difference, for in studies comparing multisensory instruction to an alternative remedial approach, the competing variables have not been well controlled.

There are in fact some practitioners who question the application of multisensory methods with all disabled readers. Doris Johnson and Herman Myklebust of the Institute for Language Disorders at Northwestern University, for example, caution that some reading disabled children appear prone to sensory overload; thus the involvement of another sensory modality may serve only to confuse them (Johnson and Myklebust 1967). Unfortunately, these clinicians have not provided empirical data to support this contention, nor have they described in detail the children they have in mind. In my opinion, it stands to reason that we should use discretion in using multisensory methods: a child with a handwriting disorder (dysgraphia), for example, will find kinesthetic activities extremely challenging at first, and it may take some time before these activities can be incorporated in his or her instructional regime; a hyperactive child having a reading disability will be more distractible than a dyslexic child without attention deficits but once familiarized with the procedures, should benefit from the additional structure and reinforcement of kinesthetic input.

Susan Bryant (1979) has compared the effects of VA (visual, auditory) with VAKT procedures on reading disabled children, keeping all other instructional variables constant. In doing so, she found no differing effects due to treatment between methods on either reading or spelling performance, despite the fact that the VAKT procedures demanded more student engaged time. However, because the intervention time in Bryant's study was only six days, efforts to generalize her results to actual clinical or classroom practice should be restrained. Conclusions drawn from one-shot experimental training studies such as Bryant's are always open to question.

After conducting an extensive review of the research on multisensory training, Bryant (1979) suggests two possible effects of multisensory instruction that are not sensitive to experimental manipulation and therefore may have gone undetected in the research thus far. The first is that multisensory methods may provide more feedback to the teacher and the child in initial learning, and the second is that multisensory activities allow for distributed and varied practice, thereby minimizing boredom.

Perhaps the most interesting research to date on the effects of multisensory instruction is that conducted by Charles Hulme. Hulme (1981), seeking to understand the rationale for multisensory instruction with disabled readers by investigating the effects of tracing on visual recognition, finds that tracing letters significantly enhances the ability of disabled readers to remember letters they have seen and brings their recognition performance up to that of normal readers who have merely been shown the letters; however, tracing has little improvement effect on normal readers. With abstract shapes on the other hand, tracing benefits both normal and disabled readers, and to a similar extent. Hulme maintains that these findings suggest that good readers have access to a phonological code, which is more efficient for storing verbal material than a visual code. In contrast, poor readers rely on visual memory which may be enhanced by kinesthetic input, such as tracing. Although this hypothesis appears to offer an explanation as to why multisensory teaching might benefit dyslexic students, the fact that tracing in Hulme's experiments improved recognition of individual items only, but not of the sequences in which the items were presented, weakens, but does not totally invalidate, the credibility of this explanantion. As Hulme himself points out, learning to read is dependent upon learning to recognize sequences of letters in words.

In attempting to understand the mechanisms underlying the effects of tracing on visual recognition, Hulme offers two competing hypotheses: (1) that tracing serves to direct attention to the stimuli to be remembered; (2) that tracing increases the information about the stimuli that may be stored in memory. Hulme questions the plausibility of the attentional hypothesis, citing the failure of similar attention-directing activities in previous research, such as haptic inspection of three dimensional objects, to enhance visual memory. Opting for the latter hypothesis, Hulme suggests that the primary effect of tracing is to provide information in memory about the movements made in tracing and posits the existence of a separate motor memory system which acts in conjunction with visual memory of the shapes of the items to be remembered. Lending support to this contention are Hulme's findings that visual interference during the experimental procedure disrupted memory for visually presented shapes but not for shapes that had been traced, whereas motor interference was most disruptive for recognition of shapes that had been traced.

Hulme asks a question more relevent to reading than the research he conducted on visual memory: Does tracing enhance memory for verbal labels of visual configurations? In a study conducted with normal-reading children, in which triplet shapes were paired with high frequency, high imagery nouns, Hulme found that names were better remembered for the triplets that had been traced. He emphasizes the implications of these resic sults for beginning and remedial reading instruction which involves a similar form of visual-verbal paired-associate learning.

Unfortunately, Hulme has not replicated this study with disabled readers, though he suggests that this be done. Moreover, although he provides persuasive evidence of the facilitative effects of tracing on verbal learning, Hulme does not identify the underlying mechanisms that produce these effects.

Whether or how information processed in one sensory modality can enhance the processing of information in another modality remains to be seen. Yet Hulme's hypothesis that multisensory processing establishes multiple memory traces that reinforce retention of information about spelling patterns has appeal. Additionally, his conjecture that the benefits gained by disabled readers but not good readers from letter tracing are attributable to "their failure to employ a speech code to memorize letters" (Hulme 1981) is extremely credible in light of what we know about the phonological coding deficits in dyslexics.

I have devoted considerable attention to multisensory instruction in this chapter because it plays a large role in so many of the existing reading and spelling programs for dyslexic children. We have ample evidence that these programs work; furthermore, practitioners using these programs appear to be highly supportive of multisensory instruction. Personally, I believe that multisensory methods, applied judiciously, with learner characteristics always in mind, can facilitate the acquisition and retention of letter-sound correspondences and spelling patterns. However, if we in the reading disabilities field are to continue to advocate multisensory techniques, we should be able to substantiate their relative contribution to the effective treatment of dyslexia. Toward this end, research efforts such as those of Hulme, need to be encouraged.

MODALITY SPECIFIC INSTRUCTION

Although the question of sensory modality preferences among reading disabled children seems closely related to the issue of multisensory training, it derives from a different theoretical perspective. Efforts to adapt instructional treatments to individual learners became prevalent in the 1960s, as information processing theory gained prominence in educational psychology. Helmer Myklebust and Doris Johnson, leaders in this movement, maintained that there are two types of dyslexic individuals, one type suffering from visual perceptual deficits, the other type from auditory processing deficits (Myklebust and Johnson 1962). Johnson and Myklebust (1967) recommended that visual dyslexics be taught by a synthetic phonics approach and auditory dyslexics by a whole-word or sight approach.

However, aptitude-treatment-interaction (ATI), as modality specific instruction came to be called, began to lose credibility as a viable concept during the 1970s, as accumulating research failed to demonstrate its effectiveness. Helen Robinson conducted an often cited study in which she tested 448 children after matching them for modality preference with either a phonics or sight approach to reading acquisition; she found neither method to be more effective with those children having the most notable differences in modality strengths (Robinson 1972). Two comprehensive ATI literature summaries (Cronbach and Snow 1976; Turner and Dawson 1978) have concluded that modality preference is not strongly related to achievement, teaching approach, or reading. As explanation for these findings, Sally Lipa, in an journal article on reading disability and its treatment, suggests,

> . . . modality teaching failed to account for the fact that, regardless of mode of presentation, words must be learned linguistically, notably in the dominant language hemisphere. Teaching in a visual manner could not obviate auditory processing of words. (Lipa 1984).

Increasing Phonological Awareness

Efforts to incorporate training in phonological awareness into reading readiness instruction are the logical extension of the widely accepted tenet that phonics knowledge is essential for reading acquisition. As Joanna Williams explained:

> If the central task of the beginning reader is seen as learning to identify and use the correspondences between letter and sound, then phonemic analysis and blending are two fundamental component skills. To identify the correspondences it is necessary to be able to isolate the units, both in orthography and in the sound stream, such that the appropriate mappings between orthography and sound can be made. (Williams 1986a).

The fact that dyslexic children have particular difficulty developing phonics skills, in addition to the accumulating evidence that they lack phonological awareness (Bradley and Bryant 1985; Fox and Routh 1980, 1983; Mann 1984; Mann and Liberman 1984), suggests that they may need preliminary training in phonological competency before formal reading instruction begins.

MEASURING PHONOLOGICAL AWARENESS

Several tests were developed in the early 1970s to measure phonemic awareness, each differing somewhat in format and materials.

Charles and Pat Lindamood have developed a procedure in which colored blocks are manipulated by students to represent sounds heard in words. The validation study for this test, subsequently called the *Lindamood Auditory Conceptualization (LAC) Test* (Lindamood and Lindamood 1979), reveals a strong correlation between test scores and word reading ability on the Wide Range Achievement Test with students from kindergarten through twelfth grade (Calfee, Lindamood, and Lindamood 1973).

Isabelle Liberman and her colleagues designed a task that required children to tap out the number of syllables or phonemes heard in words (Liberman et al. 1974). First graders' scores on this segmentation task are found to relate significantly to reading achievement in second grade.

A different task, devised by Jerome Rosner, involves deleting sound segments in words, for example, "Say 'mat' without the /m/." Significant correlations between test performance and scores on the Stanford Achievement Test are evidenced at seven grade levels, kindergarten through sixth (Rosner and Simon 1971). Subsequent to this study, Rosner developed his *Test of Auditory Analysis Skills (TAAS)* which uses a deletion task to assess auditory segmentation ability (Rosner 1975). The easier items on this test require segmenting two-syllable words, for example, "Say 'cowboy'. Now say it again, but don't say 'boy'." The most challenging items require segmenting phonemes within consonant blends: "Say 'smack'. Now say it again, without the /m/."

As I mentioned in Chapter 1, many tasks are used to test or teach phonemic awareness. Nancy Lewkowicz identifies as many as ten: sound-to-sound matching; word-to-word matching; recognition of rhyme; isolation of a beginning, medial, or final sound in a word; phonemic segmentation, or separately articulating the individual sounds in a word in correct order (commonly referred to as "sounding out"); counting the phonemes in a word; blending individual sounds to make words; deleting phonemes in words; specifying which phoneme has been deleted; and phoneme substitution (Lewkowicz 1980). As Lewkowicz observes, these tasks are not equal in ease of execution; isolating initial sounds in words, for example, is easier than isolating either medial or final sounds. In attempting to evaluate these tasks in terms of their contribution to beginning reading, Lewkowicz concludes that segmentation and blending are the two basic phonemic awareness tasks that should be included in prereading instruction. In her opinion, several of the tasks, for instance counting phonemes without pronouncing them as in the Liberman study (Liberman et al. 1974) are more difficult than segmenting and blending. The usefulness of other tasks, such as rhyming, is somewhat equivocal. However, isolating the initial phoneme appears to be a useful task in that it contributes to segmentation ability.

Despite the fact that many of these tasks have been shown to correlate with reading achievement, they may be tapping different aspects of phonological awareness according to Stanovich, Cunningham, and Cramer (1984). Therefore, it is necessary to make direct comparisons between these tasks and to measure their degree of convergence. Much like Lewkowicz, Stanovich and his co-workers have examined ten phonological tasks performed by kindergarten children. Although not identical, there is considerable overlap between their tasks and those in the Lewkowicz study. Three of the tasks that involve rhyme (substitute initial consonant, rhyme supply, and rhyme choice) do not correlate highly with the other seven phonological tasks and furthermore are found to be significantly easier than any of the other tasks. This finding, the investigators suggested, accounts for the fact that rhyming tasks are poor predictors of later reading achievement. The other seven tasks are strongly interrelated; however, "strip initial consonant" is the most difficult, too difficult, the investigators conclude, for many kindergarten children. It is worth adding that all seven measures correlate more strongly with first-grade reading achievement than does a standardized IQ test.

Stanovich et al. (1984) called the present lack of knowledge about the relative ease of execution, construct validity, or predictive validity of the various phonological tasks that have been designed, "the current Achilles' heel of phonological awareness literature." We do indeed have much yet to learn about phonological awareness and how it relates to reading, as I pointed out in Chapter 1. Until we know more about the relationship of the various phonological tasks to reading, we should be extremely cautious about using these tasks as predictive indices of reading ability, particularly in educational placement.

TRAINING IN PHONOLOGICAL AWARENESS

One of the first procedures designed to promote phoneme awareness is that of D. B. Elkonin of the Soviet Union. In *the Elkonin method,* phonemes in words are represented by a series of connected squares presented beneath line drawings of the words. As the student slowly articulates a word, he moves a counter into the square corresponding to the phoneme being pronounced. Elkonin reports that children master phoneme analysis within a short time with this method (Elkonin 1973), although no empirical data are available on his work. It is worth mentioning, however, that Eileen Ball and Benita Blachman, working in two inner-city schools in New Haven, Connecticut, used the Elkonin method for initial training in a code-emphasis program which they designed for low-achieving first-graders; follow-up achievement data on these students suggested that the intervention program was remarkably successful (Ball and Blachman 1987).

At least six major training studies have been conducted on phonological awareness within the last fifteen years. That of Charles and Pat

Lindamood (described in Chapter 13) was the first. The Lindamoods have called their program *Auditory Discrimination in Depth (ADD)* (Lindamood and Lindamood 1975). The distinguishing feature of this program is the emphasis placed on the physical aspects of sound production. The instructor focuses the attention of the student on "the oral-motor" feeling as the sound is uttered (Howard 1982). Descriptive labels referring to mouth action are provided for the different sound categories. The effectiveness of Lindamood training, as administered to all first graders, was evaluated in one elementary school over a five-year period; average reading scores for this period in grades two through five rose from the 52nd percentile to the 85.7th percentile (Howard 1982).

Jerome Rosner and Dorothea Simon trained four- and five-year-old children to add, omit, substitute, and rearrange phonemes in orally presented words and found improvement in the children's ability to deal with initial phonemes (Rosner and Simon 1971). A later study done with non-reading first graders, found significantly better reading performance after 14 weeks for those children who received *Rosner's auditory analysis training,* as compared to those who did not (Rosner 1974).

Richard Venezky's Pre-Reading Skills program (Venezky 1976), designed for kindergarteners considered to be at risk for reading failure, includes two phonological awareness components, and three visual readiness units. Children are presented with phoneme sounds in isolation and taught to associate them with animals or objects that produce those sounds, for example, a dripping faucet for *s-s-s;* an angry cat for *f-f-f.* The second auditory unit teaches blending. Venezky reports that children thus trained learned to blend phonemes, as well as to associate phonemes with objects.

Michael and Lise Wallach, after determining that disadvantaged inner-city kindergarteners had more difficulty distinguishing and manipulating phonemes than middle class children, developed a readiness program for these youngsters, using parents as tutors (Wallach and Wallach 1979). Preliminary training involves teaching phoneme recognition by having children isolate initial consonants in orally presented words. Later training is similar to the traditional synthetic phonics approach: individual letter sounds are taught in isolation; these are blended into simple words; prior to reading, all new words are analyzed phonemically. Post-testing after 30 weeks showed significant improvement in both word recognition and sentence reading for the group of children who received this training, as compared to a control group. Wallach and Wallach maintain that knowledge of phonological regularities helps these children to distinguish orthographically irregular words.

Joanna Williams' ABD (analysis, blending, decoding) reading program was developed specifically for remedial intervention within schools for children classified as learning disabled, with an emphasis on efficiency and cost effectiveness (Williams 1980). It begins with auditory syllable analysis, followed by phoneme analysis with only nine phonemes, using an adaptation of Elkonin's (1963) method. Then the phonemes, represented by wooden squares, are blended into bigrams and trigrams, and the child learns to identify the phoneme sounds within these words. Later, letter names are introduced on squares and the child manipulates the squares to make different words. Six additional letters were eventually added onto the original nine; practice on various word patterns, for example, CVC; CCVC; CCVCC[1], is given. Williams reports significantly greater improvement in phoneme analysis and blending skills for the experimental groups over the control groups. Even more important, according to Williams, is the fact that the children who received training in her study were significantly better at decoding nonsense words than the children who served as control subjects, indicating that they were able to transfer their skills to unfamiliar material.

More recently, Lynette Bradley and Peter Bryant undertook a study of phonological awareness training in England (Bradley and Bryant 1985) with six-year old children determined not to be at risk for reading failure. The training involved practice in what they called *sound categorization,* which requires the children to select out words (actually pictures of words) that differ in sound from the other three or four words in a set. Two of the activities are considered *rhyming tasks:* finding the word with a differing end sound, for example, bun, *hut,* gun, sun, and finding the word with a differing middle sound (*hug,* pig, dig, wig). The third activity is considered an *alliteration task:* finding the word that begins with a different sound (bun, bus, *rug,* bud). Training took place in forty sessions over a two year period. The sixty subjects in this study were divided into four groups. Two groups were given sound categorization tasks: one group worked only with pictures; a second group, in the first year had the same training as the first, but in the second year was given plastic letters along with the pictures and taught to form the words in the pictures, one at a time, changing only the one or two letters which made the difference. A third group, which served as a control, was taught to categorize words according to concept (animals, kitchen utensils, etc.), and a fourth group received no training at all. Bradley and Bryant report that at the end of two years, the children receiving sound categorization training scored significantly higher on standardized reading and spelling tests than the children receiving concept categorization training or those receiving no training at all. Moreover, the children who had been trained with *plastic letters* did far better than the children trained only with pictures.

This latter finding leads to a question currently asked by researchers who support the notion of phonological awareness training, i.e.,

---

[1]C = consonant; V = vowel

whether or not letters should be used in the training. William Hohn and Linnea Ehri compared training kindergarten children with letters to training them with tokens. They conclude that the former produces superior sound segmenting ability, as well as better blending skills on trained words (Hohn and Ehri 1983). On the other hand, Joanna Williams, who had children begin with squares and then move to letters in her ABD program, has offered what I believe to be sound advice. She suggests that the optimal choice of stimulus materials may depend on characteristics of the learner; dyslexics and other at-risk children, who often suffer from information overload, may respond better when letters are not involved in initial training.

It should be clear by now that phonological awareness training is in its formative stages. There is little agreement on which specific phonological skills should be taught or how they should be taught, just as there is little consensus on which measures of phonological awareness might be reliable predictors of reading achievement. Additionally, there is considerable confusion in the use of terms, such as rhyme and alliteration, across research studies and in the types of tasks chosen to represent particular phonological skills. For example, the fact that Stanovich and his colleagues (Stanovich et al. 1984) determined rhyming ability to be a poor predictor of later reading achievement appears to contradict Bradley and Bryant's claim that rhyming ability correlates strongly with later reading and spelling achievement. Are these differing conclusions due to variations in the rhyming tasks given to subjects, variations in subject characteristics, variations in the way the studies were conducted or some combination of these factors? Certainly, further research is needed to answer these questions.

This discussion of the unresolved issues surrounding phonemic awareness (also referred to as *linguistic awareness, linguistic insight,* and *metalinguistic awareness*) is intended to urge practitioners to use caution in selecting measures to test or methods to teach phonological awareness. It is not meant to discourage them from doing so, but rather to urge them to exercise judgment in making their selections. Several well designed longitudinal studies are under way that address issues related to phonological awareness. These research projects include a four-year study by Bruce Pennington at the University of Colorado, aimed at identifying phonological processing deficits that may be precursors of reading disability; a three-year training study in phonological awareness with beginning kindergarteners followed through second grade, led by Susan Brady at Haskins Laboratory; and a two-year study of the effects of instruction of phonemic segmentation with kindergarteners on their reading acquisition over a two year period, undertaken by Benita Blachman and Eileen Ball at Syracuse University.

Phonics Instruction

Among reading theoreticians today, there is almost unanimous agreement that phonics instruction should be part of the reading curriculum for all school children (Anderson et al. 1984; Chall 1983a; Liberman 1984; Resnick 1979; Venezky and Massaro 1979; Williams 1985). Furthermore, despite the fact that the research on effective reading methods has been fraught with methodological problems (Pflaum et al. 1980), the general findings suggest that early and direct teaching of sound-symbol relationships produces better decoding skills than later and less explicit phonics instruction (Chall 1983a). Since decoding ability has been shown to contribute to reading comprehension (Gough and Tumner 1986; Lesgold and Resnick 1982; Perfetti and Roth 1981; Stanovich, Cunningham, and Feeman 1984), phonics instruction seems pedagogically justified. Unfortunately, as I indicated in Chapter 1, this conclusion has not generalized broadly to classroom practice where basal reader programs predominate. Most basal programs place emphasis on teaching whole words; children are expected to apply knowledge from learned words to new words, thus learning by analogy.

The failure to teach the phonological features of the alphabet systematically is particularly detrimental to dyslexic children who seem not to acquire phonics knowledge naturally nor to apply phonological strategies spontaneously (Gough and Tumner 1986; Olson et al. 1985; Liberman et al. 1983; Mann 1986; Perfetti 1985a; Vellutino 1983). Among reading specialists who work with dyslexic children and are aware of these deficiencies, phonics instruction is fundamental (Bateman 1979; Cox 1984; Enfield 1976; Liberman and Shankweiler 1979; Slingerland 1971). However, it is important to specify how phonics should be taught to these children. Two distinct alternative approaches exist: the *explicit phonics* approach (also termed synthetic phonics instruction or the alphabet method) and the *analytic phonics* approach (also referred to as the "functional," "incidental," or "intrinsic" approach). Explicit phonics instruction, as the name implies, explicitly teaches individual grapheme-phoneme correspondences before blending them to form syllables or whole words. In contrast, the analytic approach introduces whole words first and encourages children to deduce letter-sound relationships as they appear in those words; it differs from the basal method only in that the words presented are selected for their phonemic elements which are introduced systematically, rather than for their prevalence in children's vocabularies.

Although most remedial specialists espouse the synthetic or explicit phonics approach, some theorists contend that it places undue demands on sound blending abilities, which are especially weak in dyslexic children (Lyon 1985; Olson, et al. 1985; Siegel 1985; Vellutino and Scanlon 1986). This contention should not be ignored, but unfortunately, to date, none of the studies intended to support it can be considered methodologically acceptable comparisons of an analytic versus a synthetic approach to phonics instruction with dyslexic children.

Despite the possible lessening of blending difficulties, there is reason to question the effectiveness of an analytic approach with dyslexic students. Analytic training methods, as Joanna Williams observes (Williams 1985), have proven least successful with slow learners. A training study conducted with normal and dyslexic fifth-grade students found that the latter group needed extensive training in generalizing, as well as in analogy strategies, in order to produce analogue words for nonsense words (Wolff, Desberg, and Marsh 1985). Another important point that needs to be made is that an analytic approach, to be used effectively, necessarily requires extensive reading in order to develop a broad basic knowledge of exemplar words against which to compare newly encountered words. The very fact that dyslexics read less than normally achieving students would seem to put them at a disadvantage in applying analytic decoding strategies. These caveats, in addition to the evidence that dyslexics do not spontaneously learn the phonological code, are persuasive reasons to recommend explicit phonics instruction for most dyslexic students, albeit with provision for extensive blending practice. We must recognize, however, that real and lasting gains will not be made quickly, and that accommodation for frustration and occasional disappointment should be built into instruction.

Whether or not whole words, other than irregular words, should be directly taught to dyslexic students has been debated among reading theorists. John Guthrie (1978) as well as Frank Vellutino and Donna Scanlon (1986), maintain that both *sight recognition training* and phonics instruction should be included in remedial intervention. Some remedial programs, such as the Slingerland, provide for a dual approach. Vellutino and Scanlon (1986) claim that teaching both sight and phonic strategies leads to the flexible application of these strategies in reading. They also emphasize that children seem to learn what they are taught, a point also made by Robert Calfee and Dorothy Piontowski (1981) after observing beginning readers in the classroom.

EXPLICIT PHONICS INSTRUCTION
ORTON-GILLINGHAM APPROACH

The *Orton-Gillingham approach* mentioned in Chapter 3 (page 48), was designed for *one-to-one instruction*. In 1960, Anna Gillingham and Bessie Stillman published an instruction manual for remedial teachers (*The Orton-Gillingham Approach to Remedial Training for Children with Specific Disability in Reading, Spelling, and Penmanship*), along with a small number of instruction materials. Since then, the method has become the basic model upon which multisensory remedial intervention programs for dyslexic children have been built.

June Orton, the wife of Samuel Orton, summarized the three most important distinguishing features of the Orton-Gillingham approach as follows:

1. It is a *direct* approach to the study of phonics, presenting the sounds of the phonograms orally as separate units and *teaching* the process of blending them into syllables and words for recognition in reading and recall in writing.
2. It is an integrated, total language approach. Each unit and sequence is established through hearing, speaking, seeing, writing it. Auditory, visual, and kinesthetic patterns reinforce each other and this also provides for individual differences among the students. It is a circular, multi-sensory process.
3. It is a systematic, step-by-step approach, proceeding from the simpler to the more complex in orderly progression in an upward spiral of language development. (Orton 1964, p. 11).

As Gillingham and Stillman (1960) described it, the method is built on the close association of visual, auditory, and kinesthetic aspects of language to form what they called "the language triangle." In strong contrast to an analytic phonics method, the Orton-Gillingham approach teaches letter sounds and the blending of these sounds into words. It should never be used, according to its authors, as a supplement to sight or basal reader approaches. Furthermore, any reading outside of Orton-Gillingham materials is forbidden. Complying with this restriction obviously presents a problem, and tutors using this method have had to deviate to some extent from the authors' precept with any dyslexic child who remains in a regular classroom. Gillingham and Stillman placed considerable emphasis on the need for older children to "break old habits." In order to *establish the alphabetic principle* among these children, words must no longer be viewed "as ideograms to-be-remembered as wholes" (Gillingham and Stillman 1960), and all guessing must be eliminated.

In the Orton-Gillingham approach, letters or phonograms are introduced as visual symbols printed on cards. First, the letter name (or names, in the case of digraphs) is taught: the teacher says the name, the child repeats; the teacher asks what letter it is, and the child gives the name. When this is secure, the letter sound is taught in the same manner. The association between visual and auditory characteristics of letters is made in this way. Then *auditory-to-auditory* association is established—the teacher says the letter sound and asks the pupil for the letter name. This is followed by *visual-kinesthetic* and *auditory-kinesthetic* associations. The teacher writes the letter, carefully explaining its formation and orientation, and the student traces the letter, then copies it, then writes it from memory, and finally writes it from memory with eyes averted. This last step will internalize the visual and kinesthetic image of the letter. For auditory-kinesthetic reinforcement, the teacher gives the letter sound and asks the student to write the letter that makes that particular sound. When writing, however, the student always says the letter name, not the sound, a procedure that has been called *simultaneous oral spelling (SOS)*.

The introduction of letters and letter combinations is carefully sequenced. Initially, ten letters are taught: two vowels (*a, i*) and eight consonants (*f, h, b, j, k, m, p, t*). Each is introduced with a *key word*, for example, *i*-indian. The difference between vowels and consonants is taught, drawing the student's attention to the open and closed positions of the mouth in pronunciation, and reinforced using different colored cards for vowels and consonants. These cards are used to bring learning to mastery in drill exercises. Once letter name and letter sound knowledge is secure, reading begins. Three letter cards are laid out (for example, b-i-t), and the student is asked to produce each sound in succession, repeating them with increasing speed and smoothness until able to pronounce the word. To avoid the interference of the *schwa* sound when pronouncing consonants in isolation, the student is encouraged to pronounce the first two letters together. The same associations are established with words as with letters; the child *traces, copies, and writes* each word. Printed cards for each word, provided in a file box referred to as the Jewel Case, are used in word recognition drill exercises. *Recognition speed* is encouraged through use of a stopwatch or egg timer, and the teacher keeps a progress graph for words learned. In this way, the student builds his reading lexicon.

Orton-Gillingham lessons are intended to be conducted within forty to sixty minute periods. A guide for developing a daily routine is provided in the teacher's manual. New phonograms are introduced gradually, usually not more than two in one lesson, and must be taught in invariant order to match the word cards and other materials provided. The rationale for this order is based on experience rather than research. The digraph *ch,* for instance, is taught before the letter *c* because *c* has two sounds. Easily confusable letters, such as *b* and *d,* are introduced at considerable distance in time, unless the pupil has already encountered these letters, in which case the contrasting features of the letters are emphasized. For this reason *wh* is taught along with *w* to emphasize the sound difference which is difficult for some children to discern.

In the Orton-Gillingham approach, reading of text begins only when the student is able to read c-v-c (consonant-vowel-consonant) words "perfectly" (presumably to a highly automatic level), as well as phonetic four letter words with digraphs. Stories containing words the student has learned are printed in the teacher's manual. Nonphonetic sight words, which the student has not previously encountered, are underlined and told to the student by the teacher. The student reads each sentence silently first, asking for help if needed. In *oral reading,* he is encouraged to read with inflection, although no attention is paid to word meaning or comprehension. Gillingham and Stillman contended that the pleasure children derive from finally being able to read justifies the bland contents of these texts. The same stories are used for dictation exercises.

Syllabication is taught to all students and particularly encouraged for those who previously used a whole-word approach. Practice begins with students reading words with syllables separated, followed by their rearranging jumbled syllables to form real words. They are taught to place stress marks on accented syllables. Syllable knowledge bears directly on the teaching of spelling rules (discussed in Chapter 8, entitled Spelling Instruction).

Gillingham and Stillman considered *dictionary skills* to be an essential component of language proficiency. Thus an entire chapter in the teacher's manual is devoted to teaching these skills.

Additionally, the Orton-Gillingham approach describes the evolution of written language. As an introduction to remedial instruction, the dyslexic student is given a brief history of the development of written language, from pictographs to ideographs to alphabets, which helps him to understand the concept of an alphabetic system. For teachers, a brief history of the English language is provided to increase their understanding of word derivations in our language. The information is intended to help teachers develop a knowledge of spelling patterns, and thereby transfer this knowledge to their students. No emphasis is placed on word meaning.

TEACHER TRAINING IN THE ORTON-GILLINGHAM APPROACH

Massachusetts General Hospital in Boston for many years has provided training in Orton-Gillingham instruction in an all-year program held several times a week. More recently, two seven-week summer training programs for teachers have been established, one at The Carroll School in Lincoln, Massachusetts, another at Pine Ridge School in Williston, Vermont. Additionally, the Orton Dyslexia Society sponsors workshops in Orton-Gillingham instruction at its various branches throughout the country.

EVALUATION OF THE ORTON-GILLINGHAM APPROACH

Although it has been practiced extensively with dyslexic children and adolescents, little research has been conducted to validate the effectiveness of the Orton-Gillingham approach, as defined by Gillingham and Stillman (1960). Probably the primary reason for the lack of systematic data collection is that the method has been used almost exclusively in tutorial, one-to-one situations and, to a large extent, in private practice. In addition, it is almost impossible to know to what extent tutors are complying with the instructions provided in the teacher's manual; in other words, how representative of the approach the tutoring actually is. Carl and Carolyn Kline did, in fact, train tutors in the Orton-Gillingham approach in their child guidance clinic, but admitted that some changes had to be made, such as using a phonetic basal reader program in conjunction with the Orton-Gillingham approach (Kline and Kline 1975).

Kline and Kline conducted a follow-up study with 92 dyslexic children who had received this instruction and compared their reading progress to that of 48 dyslexic children who had not received this instruction. The instruction provided the latter group, however, was not described. Analysis of the results of posttreatment test scores indicated that only 4.4 percent of the Orton-Gillingham subjects failed to improve, whereas 55.2 percent of the comparison subjects made no significant progress. The analysis also indicated that length of treatment was an important variable; in most cases, at least two years was necessary to effect substantial gains. Age, on the other hand, was not found to be a critical factor; older children in the Orton-Gillingham group made as much, if not more, improvement as younger children, contrary to the belief held by some that older dyslexics are less responsive to remedial instruction. Although this study does lend support for the Orton-Gillingham approach, the results must be treated with reservations because of methodological problems.

ANALYTIC PHONICS INSTRUCTION
THE GLASS-ANALYSIS FOR DECODING ONLY

The Glass-Analysis for Decoding Only method was developed by Gerald and Esther Glass (Glass and Glass 1976). Unlike the Orton-Gillingham synthetic phonics approach, the Glass–Analysis method presupposes a basic knowledge of phoneme-grapheme correspondences. The phrase "for decoding only" refers to the fact that word meaning and comprehension are deemphasized in order that complete attention be placed on analyzing the orthographic structure of words. The student is taught to recognize phonemic units within words. These units are not morphemes, but rather, single letters or *letter clusters*. The clusters are never isolated, but always shown to the student within the context of words. The authors of this method have identified 119 letter clusters and placed them in two sets of words, arranged in order of apparent difficulty. These words are called *service words,* their major purpose being to provide a medium in which "to foster perceptual conditioning for letter clusters."

Five procedural steps for the instructor to follow are listed in the Glass Analysis manual:

1. Identify the whole word and ask for the word to be repeated.
2. Give the sound(s) and ask for the letter(s).
3. Give the letter(s) and ask for the sound.
4. Take away letters and ask for the remaining sound.
5. Ask for the whole word. (Glass and Glass 1976)

The method closely resembles some phonemic training procedures described in the previous section. The teacher is advised never to separate letter blends or digraphs. A problem arises, however, with suffixes that may overlap letter clusters taught as units, as for example, the *er* in spider, a word containing the cluster *ide*. In this case the teacher is told to ask, "What letters say 'sp'? What letters say 'ider'? What letters say 'ide'?" and then to ask for the sounds those particular letter clusters make, but to ignore the suffix *er*. The authors claim that their intent is to teach letter clusters "which can be generalized" and to avoid "esoteric linguistic concerns about the dropping of the final /e/ before adding the suffix."

The teacher is urged to work as fast as possible, because the authors believe fast response is important for habituating decoding patterns. Fifteen minutes should be allotted for each instructional session, plus additional time in the Follow Through Practice Books, which are designed for *oral at-sight reading*. In oral reading the teacher intervenes whenever a word containing a common letter cluster is missed and tells the student what letters to attend to. If it is an irregular ("Nix") word, the teacher only

---

"ong" cluster

(For every word, say the whole word and ask that the word be repeated.)

song

[From sound to letters]

[From letters to sound]

This word is *"song"*. What is the word?
•*In the word, "song"*, what letter makes the "sss" sound?
What letters make the "ong" sound?
•*In the word, "song"*, what sound does the letter /s/ make? What sound does o/n/g make?
•If I took off the /s/ what sound would be left?
•What is the whole word?

longest

[Sound to letters]

[Letters to sound]

[Combine two]

[Take off letters or sound]

•*In the word, "longest"*, what letter makes the "lll" sound? What letters make the "ong" sound? What letters make the "long" sound? What letters make the "est" sound? What letters make the "ongest" sound?
•*In the word, "longest"*, what sound does the /l/ make?
What sound does the o/n/g make?
What sound does the l/o/n/g make?
•*In the word "longest"*, what sound does e/s/t make?
What sound does o/n/g/e/s/t make?
•If I took off the l/o/n/g, what sound would I have left?
If I took off the "est" sound, what sound would be left?
•What is the whole word?

[Remember, to end off, always tell the word and ask for its repetition]

stronger

[Ask for letters first]

[Then ask for sounds]

[Take off]

•*In the word, "stronger"*, what letters make the "st" sound?
What letters make the "ong" sound?
What letters make the "rong" sound?
What letters make the "strong" sound?
What letters make the "er" sound?
•*In the word, "stronger"*, what sound does s/t make?
What sound does the o/n/g make?
What sound does the r/o/n/g make?
What sound does the s/t/r/o/n/g make?
In the word, "stronger", what sound does the e/r make?
The o/n/g/e/r?
•If I took off the s/t, what sound would be left?
If I took off the e/r what sound would be left?
•What is the whole word?

Excerpt from Teacher Guide, Glass-Analysis for Decoding Only. (Reproduced with permission from Easier to Learn, Inc., Garden City, New York. Copyright 1976.)

voices the word and has the student repeat it. Carefully chosen basal readers may also be used for this purpose.

The Glass Analysis method was not specifically designed for disabled readers, although the manual mentions its use with students with "severe learning disabilities" and recommends that they be provided with at least 15 minute instructional sessions each day, spaced at least one hour apart. In an effort to address the needs of students having, as they expressed it, "a handicapping condition affecting learning," Glass and Glass published the Easy Starts Kit (Glass and Glass 1978a) containing twelve *cluster packs* of word cards that represent some of the more basic letter clusters found in c-v-c words (*at, in, et, ad, it, an, ap, un, op, en, ab, and*). They have also provided Follow Through Practice Books for oral reading of short sentences containing these cluster words. Words appearing in these sentences that are not cluster words are termed *preview words* and are taught as sight words before the sentences are read.

Realizing that many students do not have secure letter-sound knowledge and that this knowledge is a necessary prerequisite for the Glass Analysis method, Glass and Glass developed a program to teach the alphabet, which they called Quick and Easy (Glass and Glass 1978b). The program consists of *Alphabet Cards* (one letter to a card), *Word Cards* (c-v-c words with basic letter clusters), *Mixed Letter Cards* (eight different letters on each), and a consumable student workbook, the *Program Book,* which also contains directions for the teacher. Letter identification begins at the word level: as the teacher holds up a word card, for example, "hat," she asks the students to locate the word on their workbook page. The teacher next points to the first letter *h,* says its name, and has the students say the name aloud several times. She then asks the students to circle this letter where it appears on their workbook page. The remaining letters in the word "hat" are taught in the same way. A *Letter Starter* exercise is followed by *Do-More* exercises which provide practice both in identifying letters as the teacher names them and in naming letters as the teacher points to them. Mastery tests are provided in the back of the book to be administered informally and individually.

EVALUATION OF THE GLASS ANALYSIS METHOD

A study investigating the effectiveness of the Glass Analysis method for teaching word decoding, oral reading skills, and spelling skills was conducted (Barger 1982) with 154 reading disabled children. Pre- and posttest analyses indicated gains in decoding and significant gains in spelling, which is particularly noteworthy as spelling instruction is not a component of this method. Glass Analysis training did not increase fluency or accuracy in oral reading, however. Unfortunately, because this training was provided as a supplement to a basal reading program and because there was no control group of subjects who did not receive the training, it is not possible to determine the extent to which the basal program or the Glass Analysis method contributed to the results.

Lydia Poe investigated the effects of Glass Analysis instruction, which she referred to as segmentation training, with first grade children who were unable to segment either visually or orally (Poe 1983). A control group of nonsegmenters who did not receive training was included in the study. After four weeks of instruction it was found that oral segmentation ability, but not visual segmentation or decoding ability, was enhanced for the experimental group. Poe suggested that perhaps first graders have trouble attending to visual tasks and may need more time to improve their skills in this area.

Thus the research so far on Glass-Analysis training has produced somewhat conflicting results, and more research is certainly needed. For dyslexic children, the Glass method serves no purpose until their letter-sound associations have been secured. However, once that point is reached, the Glass method can be used to increase automaticity in word recognition, as it encourages the student to look for orthographic patterns in words. My major reservation about the method is its disregard for morphemes, such as suffixes, which bear meaning and therefore play a critical role in fluent reading and comprehension of text. I do not believe that recognition of morphemes should ever be discouraged.

THE STERN STRUCTURAL READING SERIES

The Stern Structural Reading Series, developed by Catherine Stern and Toni Gould (Stern and Gould 1965), is a beginning reading program designed to promote "learning by insight" and thus might best be described as an analytic phonics method. The Stern method presents whole words and draws the child's attention to particular elements within those words. The program begins at a readiness level which teaches phonemic awareness. The child learns to listen to and distinguish the initial sounds in orally presented words. Once letter sounds are familiar, the child learns sound-symbol correspondences through the presentation of pictures representing words beginning with the letter to be taught; the letter appears next to the picture. The child says the letter sound (not the name) and then copies the letter formation. The child also learns the difference between a vowel and a consonant at this pre-reading level (a vowel can be sung—has a prolonged sound; a consonant, instead, is "blown, mumbled, or hissed," and has a clear sound only with an accompanying vowel).

In first grade, teaching begins with spoken, not written, words. The child is shown pictures representing consonant-vowel-consonant words, all having the same vowel, for example, man, cat, hat. The teacher says one of the words, emphasizing its letter sounds, but always pronouncing the initial consonant with the accompanying vowel, and the child points to the word. Then the child says the word in the same way. In the author's view,

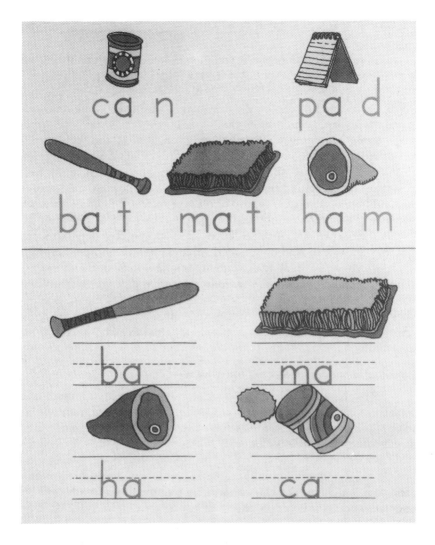

Workbook Page from Structural Reading: We Discover Reading *by Catherine Stern, Toni S. Gould, and Margaret B. Stern. (Reproduced with permission from Random House, Inc., New York, NY. Copyright 1984.)*

> The structure of the word *hat* is not revealed by adding up, in piecemeal fashion, the single elements, /h/ plus /a/ plus /t/; the word is divided structurally into a main part /ha/ and an ending /t/. The salient point in our method is this emphasis on giving the child insight into the way spoken words break naturally. (Stern and Gould 1965, p. 57)

Words for reading are color coded to emphasize the vowels and later the digraphs, final silent *e,* and suffixes. All reading is reinforced with writing (manuscript letters).

Stern and Gould stress the fact that meaning is involved at all levels of their program, first in pictures, then in individual words with picture counterparts, then in sentences, and finally in stories. Newly encountered words, such as verbs, are taught individually beforehand. Comprehension practice is incorporated at all levels.

In the beginning stages of the program, reading is discouraged in order that children do not adopt a whole word, or sight, approach before learning the individual sound-symbol correspondences. Once the basic foundations of structural analysis have been laid, Stern and Gould suggest that children be given a diversity of reading material, in addition to the readers and workbooks provided in the program. The authors contend that, in their experience, many children are so adept at sounding out words that they are able to read nonphonetic irregular words without help.

Reading and spelling are taught simultaneously in the Stern program, and reading vocabulary expands through the systematic introduction of increasingly more sophisticated common word elements. Spelling rules and "first grammatical concepts"—singular and plural noun and verb forms and simple verb tenses—are also included in the Stern curriculum.

EVALUATION OF THE STERN PROGRAM

Research on the effectiveness of the Stern program is limited, particularly in regard to its use with disabled readers. The program was developed for use in regular classrooms with children in kindergarten through second grade. Its authors, however, maintain that it is readily adaptable for remedial instruction. In the back of their book, *Children Discover Reading,* Stern and Gould provide data showing the effectiveness of their program in regular classrooms. They claim success with over one hundred students who experienced difficulty learning to read. Although they provide no empirical evidence to support this claim, they describe four successful tutoring cases, each involving a five-year-old child evidencing initial reading difficulties. It must be acknowledged that while the Stern method may be appropriate for mildly disabled readers, its utility for dyslexic children has not been verified.

In my own practice, I have used the Stern workbooks and readers selectively as a supplement to explicit multisensory phonics instruction with dyslexic elementary school students who have gained a fairly secure knowledge of sound-symbol correspondences. Children seem to like the pictures as well as the stories in these materials, which are more imaginative than most linguistically controlled text. I have found the workbook exercises to be particularly useful for demonstrating and teaching noun and verb forms and basic spelling rules.

THE MERRILL LINGUISTIC READERS

The Merrill Linguistic Readers (Fries, Wilson, and Rudolph 1966), like the Stern series, is intended as a basic beginning reading program for regular classroom use and, like the Stern, is sometimes used in remedial intervention. It also aims at teaching letter–sound correspondences within the context of real words instead of as isolated individual units. However, the Merrill program emphasizes word endings which it teaches as invariant spelling patterns (m*an, c*an, D*an,* etc.), in contrast to the Stern which presents initial consonants together with vowels (*fox, rod, hog,* etc.). The child is taught to direct his attention to word endings and to note the varying initial consonants, applying the principle of "minimal contrasts." The authors of the program maintain that

> . . . through early and continued training in perceiving minimum contrasts, the pupil will develop the habit of paying close attention to the words he is reading and will in time attain a great degree of proficiency in word recognition. (Teachers Guide for Reader Two, p. 5)

Although called a linguistic method, the Merrill approach is strongly dependent upon visual perception. Oral language activities, such as story telling and games, are suggested for children beginning the program, and the teacher is advised to make sure that pupils are aware that words are separate linguistic units by asking them to count the number of words they hear in orally presented sentences. However, no specific language stimulation materials are provided. Letter recognition is a readiness requirement. The child is taught to attend to the special visual features that identify each letter and distinguish it from others similar in shape. Letter names, but not letter sounds, are taught, and emphasis is placed on left-to-right progression.

The program, which is intended for first grade, consists of six readers and six workbooks. Before beginning each chapter, all the new *Words in Pattern* which are included in the chapter are introduced on the chalkboard, the first being c-v-c words with short *a,* as well as any high frequency words not falling in that pattern. These words are also listed in the readers. In the early books, only words with the same spelling pattern are presented together in the text, but at the more advanced level, many different patterns are juxtaposed. Pictures are excluded from all books, in order not to distract from the printed words. Pupils read the text silently first. The teacher is supposed to ask questions after every paragraph, not to check comprehension, but rather to "direct" the reading. Comprehension questions are asked at the end of each chapter; however, because of the highly controlled vocabulary and the amount of semantic redundancy, the texts are extremely bland. This limits the possibilities for meaningful discussion after reading one of the Merrill chapters, at least in the early books.

A Cat on a Mat

Is a cat on a mat?

A cat is on a mat.

Is the cat fat?

The cat is fat.

Is the cat Nat?

The cat on the mat is Nat.

Excerpt from The Merrill Linguistic Reading Program: I Can *by Rosemary G. Wilson and Mildred K. Rudolph. (Reproduced with permission from Charles E. Merrill Publishing Co., Columbus, OH. Copyright 1980).*

EVALUATION OF THE MERRILL PROGRAM

The Merrill is only one of ten or more linguistic reading programs on the market, the most widely used among them being perhaps the SRA Basic Reading Program (Rasmussen and Goldberg 1976). The basic rationale for using any of these linguistic programs with disabled readers has been that they facilitate blending, since the child does not sound out each letter. However, the linguistic approach has limited value for the dyslexic child, whose particular weakness lies in a failure to grasp symbol-sound association intuitively, because it provides no explicit instruction in grapheme-phoneme correspondences. Unfortunately, research has not yet produced empirical support for or against the use of these programs with dyslexic children. I occasionally use the Merrill materials with dyslexic students to reinforce knowledge of particular phonetic spelling patterns.

CHAPTER 6

Automaticity and Fluency

TRAINING IN AUTOMATICITY

The theory that fast, as well as accurate, word recognition is related to proficient reading was first proposed in 1974 by David LaBerge and S. Jay Samuels, as mentioned in Chapter 1. Charles Perfetti and Thomas Hogaboam in 1975 elaborated upon this hypothesis by suggesting a "limited capacity mechanism" within children's information processing systems to account for differential performance in reading comprehension. Similarly, Charles Perfetti and Alan Lesgold (1979) contend that poor decoding hampers comprehension by creating a "bottleneck"; the more time and effort required for decoding, the less processing capacity available for comprehension. Perfetti (1985a) refers to this hypothesis as a "verbal efficiency theory." Using multiple regression analysis, Keith Stanovich and his associates provide substantial support for the verbal efficiency hypothesis by determining that decoding speed is the highest contributing variable to reading comprehension (Stanovich, Cunningham, and Feeman 1984).

There is, therefore, a theoretical rationale for instruction in rapid word decoding, most particularly with disabled readers whose major weakness seems to lie in this area. Unfortunately, research so far has failed to provide direct evidence that such instruction does, in fact, improve reading comprehension. For example, Linda Fleisher, Joseph Jenkins, and Darlene Pany carried out two automaticity training studies with fourth-

and fifth-grade children who were poor readers, the first involving single words, the second involving phrases (Fleisher, Jenkins, and Pany 1979). Although such training increased the subjects' speed of single word decoding, it had no effect on their comprehension of passages containing these words. Similarly, in a training study with below average readers, Mary Strother was unable to prove that increasing speed and accuracy of word recognition directly increases comprehension of text. She concludes that subskills of reading are "mutually facilitative," that they develop through "levels of proficiency," and that "insufficiently developed subskills prevent development of higher-level "skills" (Strother 1984, abstract).

Despite the failure of experimental studies to demonstrate a causal relationship between decoding speed and reading comprehension, reading experts are paying increasing attention to automaticity training and to new methods of providing it. Recently, efforts have been made to apply computer technology toward this purpose. Such training is generally referred to as *computer asssisted instruction (CAI)*. J. F. Frederiksen and his associates have designed microcomputer activities for use with high school students who are poor readers (Frederiksen et al. 1983). These activities focus on developing three reading subskills: (1) perception of multiletter units within words; (2) efficient phonological decoding of orthographic information in words; (3) use of context frames in accessing and integrating meanings of words in context. Computer administered criterion tasks have revealed significant effects of training in the three subskill areas, as well as evidence of transfer to other componential skills of reading. As far as comprehension is concerned, the investigators maintain that increased reading speed on an inference task produces no decrement in comprehension. One of the most helpful features of the microcomputer as a training medium is its ability to provide immediate corrective feedback that can be acted upon.

Steven Roth and Isabel Beck have also investigated the effects of microcomputer automaticity training of reading subskills on reading comprehension (Roth and Beck 1984). In contrast to earlier studies with small subject samples and short-term laboratory-type intervention, Roth and Beck's training was administered in three fourth-grade classrooms over an eight-month period. A unique aspect of this training was the use of speech, provided by recordings, both for corrective feedback and assistance when needed. The major emphasis of the training was on teaching knowledge of orthographic patterns in English words. Practice conditions, intentionally designed to be semantically meaningless, forced the subjects to focus attention solely on the orthographic patterns in English words. Rapid response rates were encouraged, but for the purpose of creating a "game-like atmosphere," rather than as a means to promote better comprehension. The study comprised two principal activities, the first, called Construct-a-Word, involved subjects' constructing real words from sets of subword letter clusters; the second, called Hint and Hunt, required subjects to attend to subword letter clusters during word recognition.

Achievement tests, which measured subjects' decoding and comprehension skills relative to national norms, and laboratory tests, which measured accuracy and speed of word recognition as well as understanding of word meaning, were administered before and after treatment. Based on pretest data, subjects were split into three ability groups. Posttest analysis indicates that training benefited only those subjects in the low ability group. Almost two years gain was made on the reading vocabulary subtest of the California Achievement Test by the low ability subjects, suggesting, the investigators maintain, that decoding rather than vocabulary deficits penalize these students. Although their reading comprehension improved at the sentence level, no gains were evidenced at the passage level, paralleling findings from earlier investigations.

Roth and Beck concluded that perhaps direct training with multisyllable words not provided in their training programs was necessary to enhance proficiency with text, since many syllables that appear in longer words are not common in one-syllable words or may be pronounced differently. In addition, they caution that this type of computer instruction may not be appropriate for beginning readers who are not yet able to differentiate between real and nonsense words.

A further caution related to the use of computers with reading disabled children comes from the work of R. M. Knights (1982) who finds that the advantages of CAI for these children depends largely on the nature of the task. Although suitable for some practice purposes, computer training is not effective with reading disabled children where new learning is involved, according to Knights.

On the positive side, the potential advantages of CAI for dyslexic students are many. They include, as Judith Boettcher stipulates in an article on classroom application of computer-based education with learning disabled students: (1) provision of a one-to-one learning environment for the student, affording protection from potential embarrassment in front of the class; (2) flexibility to adjust instructional programming to individual needs, based on student responses and choices; (3) consistency of student involvement and increased time-on-task (decisions and responses on the part of the student are demanded in order for the lesson to continue, unlike normal classroom situations in which the student has the option to withdraw); (4) provision of prompt, immediate feedback; (5) practice in typing, where type-in responses are called for (which encourages accuracy and precision and discourages reversal tendencies); (6) opportunities for student decision making, such as changing the pacing or content of a lesson, by providing decision making points within programs; (7) ability to demonstrate the effects of varying one factor on the other factors involved; and (8) provision of multisensory learning experiences (typing, auditory aids, visual clues, etc.) (Boettcher 1983).

Joseph Torgesen and Kay Young stress several additional advantages of CAI activities for reading disabled students (Torgesen and Young 1984). One is that by providing a variety of formats for extensive practice or overlearning, computer-based instruction lessens the boredom that usually accompanies traditional teacher-based practice activities and hence increases sustained attention. A second important advantage is that CAI programs can accurately measure response times and, through game formats, encourage faster responses.

Computer-assisted instruction can be an expensive undertaking and, in some situations, may not pay. Therefore, those of us who are practitioners or educational decision makers must be alert to the trade-offs that may be involved in implementing such instruction. Fortunately, advances in CAI are ongoing. If we keep abreast of the relevant research literature, we will be in a better position to judge the value of newly emerging programs for the dyslexic students we teach.

TRAINING IN FLUENCY

Instructional efforts to increase reading fluency have entailed methods such as *repeated reading,* in which the student reads short meaningful passages several times until reaching a satisfactory level of fluency. Although both speed and accuracy are measured, the former is emphasized over the latter. The method is to be used as a supplement to developmental reading instruction, according to S. Jay Samuels, who is probably its leading advocate. He compares repeated reading to developing musical or athletic abilities which require practicing basic skills until they can be performed with adequate speed and smoothness (Samuels 1979).

Samuels (1986) suggests several techniques for implementing repeated reading. One technique is the *use of audio support,* where a student reads silently while listening to a tape-recorded narration of the passage. Another technique is to have the student *read for one minute and count the number of words read in that time* and then record that number on a graph; after criterion level is reached, the student moves on to another passage. *Paired reading,* having two students read alternately and record for each other the number of words read, is yet another approach.

William Henk, John Helfeldt, and Jennifer Platt suggest several additional variations of the repeated reading model, one being *imitative reading*—the teacher reads a segment of text aloud while the student follows along silently before reading the segment himself, imitating the teacher's intonation and phrasing (Henk, Helfledt, and Platt 1986). This technique is appropriate for the most disabled readers, according to Henk and his associates. *Radio reading,* in which the student, acting as announcer, reads a script aloud to the rest of the class, can avoid embarrassment, since only the student and the teacher share the script. *Chunking, or reading in phrases,* is another method suggested by these educators to promote fluency. A multisensory technique, referred to as *neurological impress* (NIM), involves the teacher and student simultaneously reading a passage aloud. The teacher forces the pace with her voice and by moving her finger along under the text, refusing to allow any pauses. Group adaption of this technique resembles the audio support method suggested by Samuels, but has not been found to be as effective as the one-to-one system, according to Henk and his colleagues.

Samuels (1986) reports on research that has shown repeated reading to be an effective instructional tool with disabled readers, particularly those with decoding problems. A theoretical explanation for this finding is proposed by Peter Schreiber, who suggests that repeated reading helps students learn to listen for the prosodic cues, such as intonation and pacing, not found in print (Schreiber 1980). Carol Rashotte investigated the question of whether repeated reading or nonrepetitive reading of passages by learning disabled students produces greater fluency and comprehension and whether degree of word overlap between passages is an influential factor (Rashotte 1983). Results of her study indicate that repeated reading is more effective than the equivalent amount of nonrepetitive reading only when there is a large number of shared words across passages.

Rashotte and Torgesen have studied the effects of *computer administered repeated reading* of passages on learning disabled fourth-grade students (Rashotte and Torgesen 1985). They find that students enjoy this activity because they receive immediate feedback on their improved reading speed and take pleasure in their ability to read the passages with increasing fluency. The major effect of this practice, however, has been to enable students to identify individual words in the passage with greater speed. Particularly encouraging is the finding that learning to read words in context seems to generalize to reading these words out of context.

Although there has been little research on fluency enhancing activities directed specifically at dyslexic students, it is my hope that more will be forthcoming, as there is certainly a place for fluency training once these students reach a sufficient decoding skill level. I should like to mention here that the Slingerland program, one of the remedial language arts programs for dyslexic children described in Part III of this book (Chapter 14), encourages fluency in round robin reading by having children first practice reading words and phrases from the chalkboard before encountering them in the basal stories.

Reading Comprehension Instruction

Dyslexic children in general receive very little training in reading comprehension (Maria 1986). For these children, reading instruction has focused almost exclusively on decoding, with minimal attention being directed toward reading for meaning. Most dyslexic children are not taught how to think or be critical when reading (Baker and Brown 1984; Harste 1985), and for most disabled readers these skills do not develop naturally. Poor readers tend to view reading as a word recognition task rather than as a process of gaining meaning from text (Canney and Winograd 1979). The problem is perpetuated by the fact that children tend to apply to their reading the particular skills or strategies they have been taught (Harste 1985). Therefore, children most needing instruction in how to comprehend text seem to be the least likely to receive it (Brown, Palinscar, and Armbruster 1984).

Reading comprehension instruction has an abysmal record, not just for reading disabled students, but for all learners. The most frequently cited evidence of this is Dolores Durkin's study in the late 1970s of reading instruction in reading and social studies classrooms (Durkin 1978–1979). Durkin and her colleagues found that out of a total of 17,997 minutes of observation, less than fifty minutes were spent on comprehension instruction. Within these fifty minutes the most frequently observed teaching behavior was the teacher's questioning students on material they had recently read. The next most common practice was the assignment of worksheets focusing on various skills. Durkin observed no instances of application, by which she meant having students apply a newly taught skill to a new example. Durkin's (1984) study of teachers' manuals in basal reading programs reveals that teacher questioning and the assignment of worksheets are the dominant instructional modes. Furthermore, where application of new skills is indicated, no prior instruction is specified. Durkin maintains that basal readers tend to teach comprehension only by implication.

Despite the fact that the last decade has witnessed a tremendous surge of interest in reading comprehension, Diane Stephens finds that out of 574 reading comprehension studies conducted in this period only thirty-seven, most of them since 1980, involved learning disabled subjects, (Stephens 1985). However, there is good reason to be optimistic, for this relatively small body of research has extremely important implications for future reading instruction with dyslexic children (Harste 1985; Maria 1986; Pearson and Gallagher 1983). Training studies carried out with poor, and in some cases disabled, readers show that these individuals can be taught the same skills and strategies that good readers have been observed to use (Pearson and Gallagher 1983).

Several comparatively new concepts have been considered in the research on reading comprehension, as Katherine Maria (1986) has pointed out. One is the importance of the *reader's background knowledge* to his understanding and interpretation of text. Awareness of this factor led to the conceptualization of *schemata,* or psychological frameworks that spontaneously develop out of an individual's cultural experience (Rumelhart 1980) (see page 12). According to this view, the reader must fit new facts from the text into his mental schema for the particular theme described in the text or, if necessary, adjust his schema.

Another concept which has had tremendous influence on reading comprehension research is *metacognition,* defined by Linda Baker and Ann Brown as "the knowledge and control the child has over his or her own thinking and learning activities" (Baker and Brown 1984). Baker and Brown refined this definition by making the distinction between knowledge (the awareness of the processing demands of a particular task) and control (the ability to check, plan, monitor, or evaluate one's own activities while reading). An additional important component of their definition of metacognition is the development and use of compensatory strategies.

A third concept that has gained prominence in the reading comprehension literature is the notion of greater *interaction between student and teacher* in the learning situation. This concept developed out of L. S. Vygotsky's theory of guided learning within a student's "zone of proximal development," which he described as

. . . the distance between the actual development level as determined by individual problem-solving and the level of potential development as determined through problem-solving under adult guidance or in collaboration with more capable peers (Vygotsky 1978).

Reuven Feuerstein's theory of *mediated learning* has also contributed to the research efforts to increase teacher-student interaction in the learning process. Feuerstein maintains that early learning is shaped by parent-child interactions and that, through interacting with adults who model and guide problem-solving activities, the child becomes able to carry out these activities on his own (Feuerstein 1979).

The three concepts just discussed—schema theory, metacognition, and mediated, or guided, learning—have led researchers to experiment with different models for teaching reading comprehension, many of which have been successful for learning disabled as well as average readers. The concepts have also inspired a new picture of the instructional conditions thought to promote optimal learning. For example, bridging the gap for the reader between his background knowledge and the information in the text is seen as an important role for the teacher (Beck, Omanson, and McKeown 1982). Although over the years there have been many suggested methods for filling this gap—for example, vocabulary training, providing advance organizers, administering pretests, including illustrations—much of the research on the effectiveness of these methods is inconclusive (Tierney and Cunningham 1984). (It is interesting to note that illustrations have been found to have a negative effect on the comprehension of learning disabled readers, but a beneficial effect on that of normal readers [Harber 1983].) A more successful approach with young, as well as at-risk, readers has been *prereading discussion* of subject matter relevent to the information in the text (Au et al. 1985; Tharp 1982; Hansen 1981).

Rather than teaching individual skills, as has been customary in most classrooms, the newer view of comprehension instruction holds that the emphasis should be placed on teaching metacognitive strategies that can be generalized across a wide variety of tasks and situations. Previous experience in teaching individual skills, such as finding the main idea or topic sentence, have been largely unsuccessful (Harste 1985). One of the major problems of the skills approach, according to Maria, is that of defining a particular skill—for example, What do we mean by main idea?—as well as deciding which of the vast number of skills presumed to foster comprehension should be taught. Jerome Harste observed that there is a subtle but important difference between skill and strategy, the former having an inflexible, obligatory connotation: "What used to be called skills should be called strategies and presented, not as mandates, but as options" (Harste 1985). Strategies are perhaps best described as *problem-solving behaviors*. Isabel Beck and Margaret McKeown make the point that many of the strategies now being labeled as metacognitive skills were formerly taught as study skills, the difference being that under the metacognitive label, the rationale for the application of these strategies is explained to students.

Linda Baker and Ann Brown offer a particularly apt description of the way guided learning theory has been applied in the "new wave" of reading comprehension instruction:

> The current interest in dynamic learning situations has seen a move away from experimenter-controlled or teacher-controlled instruction of the traditional kind towards a concentration on interactive processes. It is through interactions with a supportive, knowledgeable adult that the student is led to the limits of her own understanding. The teacher does not tell the student what to do and then leave her to work on unaided; she enters into an interaction where the child and the teacher are mutually responsible for getting the task done. As the child adopts more of the essential skills initially undertaken by the adult, the adult relinquishes control (Baker and Brown 1984, p. 382).

According to Ann Brown and her colleagues, Annemarie Palinscar and Bonnie Armbruster, "the ideal teacher functions as a model of comprehension-fostering and monitors activities largely by activating relevant knowledge and questioning basic assumptions" (Brown, Palinscar, and Armbruster 1984). Only by the teacher's relinquishing her responsibility for problem solving, does the child come to internalize the strategy (Vygotsky 1978). Harste claims that most direct instruction models, by assuming that only the teacher can teach, do not allow for internalization, nor do they provide opportunity for students to learn from their peers (Harste 1985).

Two additional perspectives differentiate the newer from the traditional approaches to reading comprehension instruction. One is that the focus of instruction has moved from an emphasis on product (defined either as gaining specific information from the text or as learning a particular skill in a specific situation) to an emphasis on process (learning how one goes about getting meaning from text). As Katherine Maria stresses, it is much more important for teachers to know how students arrive at their answers than to determine whether or not the answers are correct (Maria 1986). Ultimately, if students understand the process required, their responses will be appropriate.

The other instructional perspective that has begun to influence the teaching of reading comprehension is what Baker and Brown have termed *the contextualization of skills* (Baker and Brown 1984). Rather than relying on skill-packages to teach specific basic skills, such as summarizing, finding the main idea, sequencing facts, etc., the newer approaches "teach essential strategies in the *context* of actually reading or studying with the *goal* of arriving at a coherent interpretation of the text" (Baker and Brown 1984).

Maria provides a useful framework within which to view much of the research that has relevance for dyslexic students. She determined that essentially two basic models of comprehension instruction have developed over the last several years, both of which have been applied to students described either as "poor" or "disabled" readers: the explicit comprehension model and the text-based model.

In the *explicit comprehension approach,* attributed to David Pearson (Pearson 1982; Pearson and Leys 1985), the teacher chooses a particular strategy, such as drawing inference, and selects the reading material for teaching that strategy. She then demonstrates four steps to apply in reading the text: (1) asking a question, in this case an inferential question; (2) answering the question, which usually involves reading over the sentence or paragraph; (3) finding evidence to support the answer; and (4) explaining the reasoning process. After the teacher has modeled all four steps, she begins to turn over the problem-solving task to the students by performing steps 1 and 2 and asking the students to provide evidence for the answer and indicate their reasoning. The teacher may then ask the inferential question and point to the evidence, but ask the students to provide the answer. In the next stage the teacher will only ask the question and the students will perform steps 2 through 4. Finally, the students take responsibility for the entire sequence.

In the *text-based model,* for which Maria credits Walter MacGinitie, the teacher first chooses a particular text that she feels the students are likely to enjoy and, after reading it through carefully, decides one particular strategy or skill which might be successfully applied to this text. The instructional process in this model is essentially the same as that of the explicit comprehension model, the only significant difference being a greater emphasis on interest and motivational factors in the text-based model. Maria states, however, that many instructional studies or programs do not fit perfectly into one or the other category of her classification scheme, but may contain certain components of either or both models.

One of the more noteworthy research endeavors on comprehension instruction, and one which fits best into the explicit comprehension category, is that of Jane Hansen (1981). Using second grade students, she compared two experimental methods for teaching inferential reasoning to a control condition that followed the more typical basal reader approach. The latter included prereading activities, which Hansen did not specify, and a postreading question format consisting of eighty percent literal questions and twenty percent inferential questions.

One experimental approach derived its rationale from schema theory and entailed a unique prereading activity intended to bring the students' background knowledge to bear on the story to be read. The experimenter chose three important ideas from the story and asked the students to call up their own experience with each idea and, based upon their experience, predict what might happen in the story. To provide a concrete picture of the mental process, Hansen had the subjects in this treatment condition write down their experiences on strips of grey paper and their predictions on strips of pink paper and as a follow-up activity weave the strips together into their "brains," as she expressed it. The postreading questioning format for these subjects was the same as that for the control subjects.

In the other experimental condition, subjects followed the same procedures as the controls, except that the postreading activity consisted of 100 percent inferential questions. Ten stories were studied in this manner, each over a period of four days.

At the end of the period, several experimenter-designed tests, as well as a standardized reading test, were administered. Results across these tests were not totally consistent; however, the experimental approaches, and particularly the inferential questioning approach, tended to produce higher scores than the control treatment.

As a follow-up study, Hansen, together with David Pearson, a leading expert on reading and reading instruction, merged the strategy training and questioning practice into a single three part treatment: (1) making students aware of the importance of inference; (2) having students discuss experiences similar to text events and predict what might happen next; and (3) providing students with many inferential questions to discuss after reading the text (Hansen and Pearson 1983). Subjects in this study were fourth grade students, half of them good readers and half poor readers. Posttreatment measures, which involved reading stories and answering comprehension questions, indicated that the poor readers benefited significantly from the treatment while the good readers were bored by the instructional texts, which were written below their reading proficiency level. The important finding is that poor readers can be taught comprehension strategies and learn to apply them successfully in reading.

An especially innovative approach to strategy training with disabled readers is Annemarie Palinscar and Ann Brown's *reciprocal teaching* method, which appears to comprise some of the most effective aspects of both explicit comprehension and text-based instructional models (Palinscar and Brown 1983, 1985). The reciprocal teaching model contains two major components, the first being the four strategic pupil activities taught: generating questions about the text, summarizing the text, predicting what will happen next, and clarifying or evaluating what the students have read. The second critical component is an interactive dialogue between teacher and students and eventually among the students themselves about the text and the four strategies applied to processing the text.

Instruction begins with a teacher led discussion about the kinds of problems readers may experience in comprehending what they read. It

---

Aquanauts

Student 1: My question is, what does the aquanaut need when he goes under water?

Student 2: A watch

Student 3: Flippers

Student 4: A belt

Student 1: Those are all good answers.

Teacher: Nice job! I have a question too. Why does the aquanaut wear a belt, what is so special about it?

Student 3: It's a heavy belt and keeps him from floating up to the top again.

Teacher: Good for you.

Student 1: For my summary now... This paragraph was about what the aquanaut need to take when they go under the water.

Student 5: And also about why they need those things.

Student 3: I think we need to clarify "gear."

Student 6: That's the special things they need.

Teacher: Another word for gear in this story might be equipment, the equipment that makes it easier for the aquanauts to do their job.

Student 1: I don't think I have a prediction to make.

Teacher: Well, in the story they tell us that there are "many strange and wonderful creatures" that the aquanauts see as they do their work. My prediction is that they will describe some of these creatures. What are some of the strange creatures that you already know about that live in the ocean?

Student 6: Octopuses.

Student 3: Whales?

Student 5: Sharks!

Teacher: Let's listen and find out. Who will be our teacher?

A Reciprocal Reading Teaching Script. (Reproduced with permission from the author, Annemarie Palinscar.)

introduces the four comprehension strategies and explains why they are helpful. The discussion aims at stimulating metacognitive awareness so that students learn to guide and monitor their reading comprehension.

Focusing on a particular reading selection, the teacher models each of the four strategic activities for the students, beginning at the paragraph level (though often at the sentence level for more disabled readers). Once students have caught on, the teacher turns over her role to one of the students, who leads the activities and calls on other students (the reciprocal teaching component). The teacher subtly guides and provides feedback to the student-teacher. After the activities have been mastered with practice materials, they are applied to classroom texts.

Palinscar and Brown (1983, 1985) conducted several evaluation studies of their techniques and reported significant improvement in students' comprehension, as measured daily on reading passages. This level of improvement was maintained over eight weeks following treatment. Furthermore, training effects carried over to tests in other subject areas, such as science and social studies (Brown, Palinscar, and Armbruster 1984).

Taking a rather unique perspective on the reading process, Marian Blank investigated the effects of "non-content," or function, words on comprehension of sentences. As mentioned in Chapter 2, she determined that children have more difficulty reading and spelling words such as "is," "was," "not," "does," than content words, which by nature have higher semantic value, and she emphasized that dyslexic children have severe problems dealing with non-content words (Blank and Bruskin 1982). To make matters worse, Blank contends that non-content words are given particularly short shrift in remedial programs for disabled readers because they tend not to be spelled phonetically and most of these programs stress the phonetic regularity of English words. Non-content words are considered confusing exceptions and are usually taught in isolation as sight words with little attention to meaning.

Blank has developed a method for *teaching noncontent words* as part of the regular reading curriculum. A major priority in her instructional approach is having children attach semantic importance to these words as they appear in sentences. The semantic information provided in noncontent words often helps the reader anticipate particular features of the words that follow, for example, singular or plural forms.

To build awareness and understanding of noncontent words, Blank constructed a series of books, arranged according to sentence types and in order of difficulty. The first level teaches eight of the most frequently used noncontent words (*the, here, is,* etc.) and then presents them in the context of three basic sentence types ("Here is a boy; The boy can jump; The boy is jumping.") The second level teaches past tense with *was* and *were,* the yes-no question form, and the concepts *but* and *now,* presenting them in sentences. The third level introduces adjectives and possessives and the *ed* form of past tense verbs. The sentences in these instructional books are highly redundant, semantically explicit, and often split between pages so that students learn to anticipate the words to follow. English grammar rules are not directly taught; the intention is for students to glean rules through experience with sentences. Amusing cartoon drawings are included to entertain as well as to help convey meaning. Blank's program has been used with learning disabled children from six to twelve years of age and, according to Blank and Bruskin (1982), with apparently promising results in terms of the ability to write sentences and to comprehend text.

The recent work of Joanna Williams on *main idea identification* with learning disabled children (Williams 1986b) represents an innovative approach to one of the more traditional lines of comprehension instruction. Acknowledging that there is considerable controversy over the definition of "main idea," Williams avoids the term altogether and borrows instead the labels "general topic" and "specific topic of discourse" from Walter Kintsch and Teun van Dijk's theory of text processing, where the general topic is the title subject of an essay or story and the specific topic of discourse is the topic sentence or implicit main idea in each paragraph (Kintsch and van Dijk 1978). Williams contends that the ability to select main ideas from text requires basic classification skills; thus, she provides

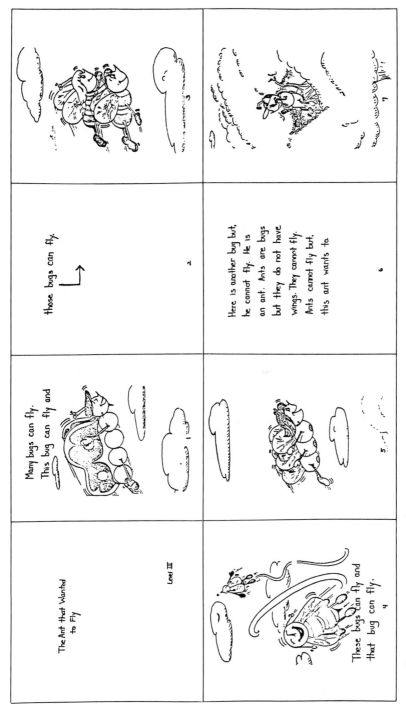

Excerpt from The Sounds of Sentences by Marian Blank. (Reproduced with permission from the author. In press.)

students with initial instruction in categorizing objects and pictures, which is later related to text organization.

When first working at the paragraph level, students are asked "What is this paragraph about?" (meaning, what is the general topic?) and then required to circle the word referring to the general topic in the paragraph. The next question asked is "Does this paragraph tell us everything about _____?" "No, it doesn't." "What is the specific topic?" In this way students learn to identify topic sentences within paragraphs. Later they learn to determine the main ideas in paragraphs that do not contain topic sentences, the more common type of paragraph found in text, according to Williams. Students also learn to identify anomalous sentences using a similar questioning procedure. All work is carefully sequenced from easy to difficult, from choosing titles, for example, to writing summaries.

Investigating the effectiveness of this approach with eleven-year-old learning disabled children, Williams found that they produced better paragraph summaries than other same-age learning disabled children who did not receive the training. However, their performance on posttests was far from optimal, leading Williams to conclude that the length of training time needs to be extended for these children.

Another approach to improving the reading comprehension of disabled readers that is beginning to be explored is to encourage the *use of mental or visual imagery* in text processing. A study conducted by a research team from The University of Kansas Institute for Research in Learning Disabilities found visual imaging to be as effective as self-questioning for enhancing the reading comprehension of six learning disabled adolescents (Clark et al. 1984). A more recent study indicates that instructing fourth- and fifth-grade poor readers to "make pictures in your mind" helped them to identify implicit, as well as explicit, inconsistencies in the passages they were asked to read (Gambrell and Bales 1986). These children were significantly more successful at noting semantic inconsistencies than were children in a control group who were asked to, "Do whatever you can to understand and remember what you read." Training in either condition was only thirty minutes.

Nanci Bell has developed a program to teach visual imagery strategies to children and adults with reading comprehension problems (Bell 1986). Bell believes strongly that imaging is necessary for integrating the information in written or spoken language and that poor readers, ". . . cannot generalize and create a whole—gestalt—from the information." The program manual, entitled *Visualizing and Verbalizing for Language Comprehension and Thinking,* provides the teacher/tutor with explicit instructions on how to take students through a series of steps in applying visual imagery to written language processing, as well as sample lesson scripts and case descriptions.

Because some people have trouble verbalizing as well as visualizing what they read or hear, training begins with *picture to picture* exercises. The student describes a given picture to the teacher and the teacher in turn tells the student what his description made her visualize ("Your words made me picture. . . ."). In this way he receives feedback about his verbalization and can make any necessary modifications. *Structure words* are provided on 3 × 5 cards to cue the student to include greater detail in his descriptions and ultimately in his own images. "Gross" structure words include *what, size, shape, number, color,* and *where.* "Fine" structure words for more subtle detail include *when, background, movement, mood, perspective* (from where the student is observing the image), and *sound.*

The next training stage, *word imaging,* starts with the student visualizing an object within his sight: looking at that object, closing his eyes and visualizing it, and then describing it. Then the student is asked to recall something familiar such as a pet, visualize it, and describe it. Bell refers to this as *personal imaging.* The third step of the word imaging stage is *known noun imaging,* where the teacher provides single words for the student to visualize and describe, such as, "airplane," "tiger," or "clown." Training moves on to *single sentence imaging.* The teacher reads a simple sentence, for example, "The cat is on the chair," and the student adds details to embellish the sentence, such as the size and color of the cat or the chair.

The *sentence-by-sentence imaging* stage is a major point in Bell's imagery program. As the teacher reads the first sentence in a paragraph, the student forms an image for that sentence, verbalizes the image, using the structure words to cue details, and then places a 3-inch felt square on the table to "anchor" that sentence image. The process is repeated with the sentences that follow. The felt squares are placed vertically, one beneath the other, to reinforce the concept that the sentences build on each other. After the student is able to do this with some proficiency, he is given sentences to read aloud and then sentences to read silently. Bell suggests published materials that are useful for these purposes. Later in this stage, the student is asked to give a picture summary of the sentences in the paragraph, a word summary, and a main idea for the paragraph. The teacher begins to ask interpretive questions that reflect the taxonomy of reading comprehension skills: inferring, predicting, concluding, and evaluating.

Multiple sentence imaging (visualizing and describing information in several sentences together) is actually a pared down version of the previous stage in that some of the steps are removed; for example, felts are optional and structure word cards are no longer used. Reaching this stage may take some time, as imaging should now be fairly automatic. The remaining stages of the training progression are *whole paragraph imaging,* followed by *paragraph-by-paragraph imaging,* and finally *whole page imaging* (integrating information from several paragraphs into visual images).

Though designed essentially for one-to-one tutorials, Bell has provided suggestions for its use with small groups. For example, one student does the imaging and the other students take turns in taking the teacher's role. Bell has not conducted group studies with her program, though she has many individual case studies that attest to its effectiveness.

While imagery may play a facilitative role in reading comprehension, there are several potential drawbacks to be considered when encouraging visual imagery as a comprehension strategy. The first is based on the well recognized fact that there is tremendous variation in the degree to which people use visual imagery to process language. Although Bell has implied that anyone can be taught to visualize, there is no reliable evidence to support this claim. It may be that for some people imaging is antithetical to their cognitive style. For example, a highly intelligent and extremely articulate psychology professor with whom I once studied told his class in a lecture on imagery that although he was a prolific reader, he was unable to visualize verbal information.

A second problematic issue is that not all written language lends itself to visual imagery. The reader must be able to judge when and when not to apply imagery strategies; dyslexic readers who have had less experience than good readers may find it particularly difficult to make this judgment. A third point to be considered is that unless imaging occurs at a highly automatic level, it may interfere rather than facilitate comprehension; at the very least it will decrease reading speed. As practitioners working with dyslexic students we need to keep these issues in mind in deciding which students might benefit from imagery training and under what conditions.

Computer-assisted instruction (CAI) has also been applied to teaching reading comprehension skills. One example of such application is the program developed by Control Data Corporation called the *Reading Comprehension System* described by Judith Boettcher (1983). The program teaches five comprehension skill areas: semantics (word meanings, as well as practice with synonyms, antonyms, and analogies), syntax, relationships (simple comparisons, as well as temporal, spatial, social, and logical relationships), inferencing, and interpretation. These skill areas are taught at five levels of difficulty and applied to short reading passages written at six vocabulary levels. This structure comprises a five-by-six matrix that enables the teacher to select appropriate comprehension exercises for students according to their levels of comprehension skill and vocabulary knowledge. All passages are followed by ten questions, two for each of the comprehension skill areas. The student types his responses—in most cases "yes" or "no"—and receives immediate feedback on the screen indicating whether a response is right or wrong. The program has a built-in mechanism for judging mastery and ceases to present questions in a skill area when mastery has been reached. In addition to a program manual, the teacher is provided with forms on which to record each student's progress and by which to determine the appropriate point for the student to reenter the program.

Boettcher conducted a study of the effectiveness of this CAI program with 28 learning disabled students in self-contained fourth- and fifth-grade classrooms. The average training time for students was forty-five minutes per week. At the end of nine weeks, comparison of pre- and posttest scores on the California Achievement Test indicated that these students had made on average approximately a year's gain on vocabulary and reading comprehension subtests. Boettcher acknowledges that there is considerable variance in the amount of gain among students; that nine students were not available for posttesting; and that, in absence of a control group, pre- and posttest gain scores have low reliability. Despite these shortcomings, she concluded that the gains were impressive.

There are, and undoubtedly will continue to be, further developments in the use of computers to teach reading comprehension skills. The major advantage of CAI is its provision of individualized practice in skill building within classroom settings. However, CAI is only as effective as the software programs that are designed. As practitioners and educational decision makers our major task in this regard is to learn how to evaluate the quality of these programs before investing large sums of money to implement them in schools.

One other instructional technique worth noting, although there has been no research to determine its effectiveness, is the Slingerland *phrase reading method* which is used in small group round robin reading (Slingerland 1971). In this approach, the teacher guides the students' comprehension of text by applying *wh* questions to their oral reading. It begins with the teacher asking all the students to read a sentence silently. The teacher then directs the first child to read, for example, the phrase that tells when the story takes place, and the child responds with the opening phrase, for example, "One sunny day." The next request might be to read the phrase that tells where the story takes place, and the second child would read the following phrase, for example, "on a big ranch in the West." Subsequently, who and what questions would be asked that direct the children's attention to subject and object of the sentence. Although the stated rationale for this technique is to encourage reading fluency, perhaps the greater contribution of this approach is teaching children how to process text for meaning.

CHAPTER 8

Spelling Instruction

PRINCIPLES OF SPELLING INSTRUCTION

Some of the most important pedagogical issues related to spelling instruction are brought to light by Margaret Stanback and Marylee Hansen in their review of the literature on spelling instruction (Stanback and Hansen 1980). One of these issues, which has been referred to as the "generalization controversy" (Yee 1966), concerns the question of whether or not the sound-symbol correspondence of English orthography is sufficiently regular to warrant teaching rules and regularities. This question has provoked a number of studies aimed at determining the amount of regularity in the English spelling system. Ernest Horn, the staunchest opponent of teaching generalizations in spelling, states that over a third of the words in a standard English dictionary have more than one pronunciation, that more than half of these contain silent letters, that most sounds are spelled in several ways, that most letters, particularly vowels, have more than one sound, and that unstressed syllables are hard to spell (Horn 1960). Horn advocates teaching only those rules that apply to a very large number of words and have few exceptions. In contrast, Paul Hanna and his associates, after conducting a computerized analysis of 17,000 English words, conclude that only three percent required rote memorization, falling into the category of "demon" words (Hanna et al. 1966).

Whereas Horn and Hanna and his colleagues examined only the phonemic regularity of English words, Richard Venezky has analyzed

20,000 words, taking into consideration morphemic features as well. As a result of his findings, Venezky recommends three categories of spelling patterns: (1) predictable, (2) unpredictable and frequent, and (3) unpredictable and rare, rather than the standard two category regular/irregular classification (Venezky 1970).

Although research on the instructional implications of the generalization controversy has apparently produced ambivalent results, Stanback and Hansen cite two studies that imply that direct instruction in spelling generalization was beneficial to slower learners. They conclude that there may not be one best way to teach spelling, but observe that

> . . . in the light of analyses such as Venezky's, the phonology and orthography are seen to be closely related, especially when certain morphological principles are understood. For example, the past tense marker *ed* is consistently spelled, no matter that it is pronounced in three different ways, e.g., /id/ in *landed,* /d/ in *planned,* and /t/ in *rushed.* In fact, the morphology is highly dependable for spelling, as there are few exceptions. Prefixes and suffixes, inflectional and derivational, are added to roots by fixed and dependable rules. (Stanback and Hansen 1980)

Another important instructional issue is whether spelling should be taught *systematically,* as a relatively independent subject, or whether it is best taught *incidentally* in the context of other subject areas. Here again, there is no definitive empirical support for either approach; however, as Stanback and Hansen point out, research indicates that the hundred most frequently misspelled words are among the most frequently occurring words in text, and therefore it seems clear that repeated exposure to a word in reading does not ensure spelling knowledge of that word.

The *frequency of testing* in spelling instruction, the *type of practice* provided (distributed versus massed), and the *number of spelling words* presented in a lesson have been found to have differing effects on good and poor spellers. According to Stanback and Hansen, these variables have only minimal influence on good spellers, but poor spellers do better with frequent (daily) testing, with distributed rather than massed practice, and with fewer numbers of words per lesson.

Roderick Barron maintains that poor readers are more likely to use an orthographic approach (attending to spelling patterns) to reading and a phonological approach (attending to letter sounds) to spelling, but that good readers are able to apply either strategy as needed (Barron 1980). Therefore, he advises teaching both strategies and cautions that too much emphasis on one or the other strategy might encourage overspecialization of that strategy. However, research support for this contention, as well as for any approaches to spelling instruction, is lacking. For knowledge of effective teaching methods for dyslexic students, we are dependent on reports from practitioners working with these students (Stanback and Hansen 1980).

MULTISENSORY METHODS OF REMEDIAL SPELLING INSTRUCTION

Multisensory teaching has probably had its greatest impact in the area of remedial spelling instruction, the two best known approaches being the *Orton-Gillingham* and the *Fernald*. As previously described in Chapter 4, the *Orton-Gillingham* approach teaches spelling as the inverse of, in conjunction with, and as reinforcement for, reading. Learning progresses from small units (phonemes and syllables) to larger units (words and sentences). Enormous emphasis is placed on the alphabetic principle and phonetic regularity of the English spelling system. All learning is carefully sequenced. Inconsistent spelling patterns are only gradually introduced, and optional spelling patterns representing similar sounds are taught as separate units. Irregular spellings are not taught until the student becomes comfortable with phonetic spellings. Although considerable practice with syllables is provided, inflectional endings, as well as prefixes and suffixes, are treated as morphemes and taught by the rule. The technique applied to studying spelling is *simultaneous oral spelling (SOS)*, wherein the child pronounces the word, spells it orally, and then writes the word, saying the letter names as she writes.

In contrast to the Orton approach, the *Fernald* method (Fernald 1943), while also multisensory, teaches spelling with whole words of the student's own choosing, rather than word units following an orderly sequence. The Fernald procedure closely resembles the *neurological impress* method described on page 77. It focuses on the student's development of a distinct visual image of the word and automaticity for the motor pattern for writing the word, both processes being mutually reinforcing. The technique involves having the student say the word while looking at it with the teacher underlining each syllable as it is pronounced. The student then repeats the word slowly, tracing each syllable as it is pronounced. The next step requires the student to write each syllable while saying it slowly so that individual letter sounds may be heard. Finally the student writes the whole word from memory (while pronouncing it) on the reverse side of his paper. With some students the tracing stage may be bypassed. However, words are never copied. Fernald's approach is based on the rationale that putting all modalities into play compensates for weaknesses in visual perception and visual memory.

Another multisensory approach to spelling is *Bannatyne's method* which shares some of the features of the two methods just described while differing from them in several respects (Bannatyne 1971). Alexander Bannatyne is primarily concerned with the sound blending problems demonstrated by many learners and stresses the need for disabled spellers to hear their "phonemic vocal inner language" in order to master the sequencing aspects of spelling. Bannatyne's technique requires the student to first pro-

nounce the spelling word slowly, then to pronounce it separating the phonemes, then to study the word in print visually, separating the graphemes
representing the phonemes, then to pronounce each phoneme in sequence
as the teacher points to the corresponding grapheme, then to write the
graphemes while articulating the phonemes as a rhythmic sequence, and
finally to practice this technique until the word is learned. Tracing and
copying may be involved if necessary. Multisyllable words are introduced
only when the student can spell at the syllable level; with multisyllable
words, the syllable, rather than the individual phoneme, becomes the ar-
ticulated unit.

The Childs Spelling System (Childs and Childs 1971, 1973) is one of
several variations on the Orton-Gillingham approach to remedial spelling
instruction. Sally and Ralph Childs, the authors of this method, have reorganized and simplified many of the Orton-Gillingham generalizations
and rules, classifying spelling words into three groups: sound-words, which
can be sounded out, think-words, which require individual study, and see-
words, which require memorization. Multisensory techniques are not applied, however, in the Childs system.

The Slingerland Multisensory Approach to Language Arts for Specific
Language Disability Children (Slingerland 1971), which was developed for
classroom use, incorporates a simultaneous auditory-visual-kinesthetic approach intended "to strengthen inner sensory associations" (Aho 1967) and
begins with handwriting instruction. Students first trace, then copy, and
then write each letter formation while provided with the letter sound. After a letter formation has been mastered, students are given the letter
name, as well as a key word for the letter sound; they must then name the
letter as they write it, give the key word, and produce the letter sound.
Extensive kinesthetic input is a distinctive feature of the Slingerland
method. In spelling practice, the teacher says the letter sound or word and
students write the letter or letters in the air while saying the letter name,
the rationale being that learning will be further reinforced through engag-
ing the large, as well as the fine, motor system. In addition to tracing with
two fingers, and then with the eraser end of a pencil, writing is done initially on large spaced paper to encourage large letter formations.

Slingerland classifies spelling words into three categories. Green-
flag words, or short vowel, purely phonetic words, are studied by having
the teacher dictate the word, the student repeat the word and then give the
vowel sound. The student then names the vowel while forming it in the
air, then spells the word orally, writing each letter in the air as he names it,
and then says the word. Finally, the student writes the word on paper and
traces it with two fingers for further memory reinforcement.

In red-flag words, which are nonphonetic or irregularly spelled, the
difficult parts are stressed, but the word is studied as a whole, involving
primarily the visual and kinesthetic modalities. The student copies the

word from a model, the teacher checks spelling and letter formations, the student traces over the word, naming each letter, and then, when ready, closes his eyes and writes the word in the air.

Yellow-flag words are words containing ambiguous spelling patterns, or patterns representing sounds that can be spelled in more than one way (for example, *ai, ay, a-e, eigh* all for long /a/), and are introduced only after vowel digraphs, diphthongs, and phonograms have been taught. By third grade, students should be able to recall all of the possible spellings for phonograms and to select the correct one for particular words (Aho 1967). Considerable practice with morphographs, syllables, and spelling rules is provided in the Slingerland program. All learning is reinforced by writing from dictation, first at the letter, then the word, and then the sentence level.

In *Alphabetic Phonics,* Aylett Cox incorporates the Orton-Gillingham principles but has reorganized the Orton spelling generalizations and rules (Cox 1984). She brings spelling instruction to a considerably more complex and sophisticated level, as is reflected in the subtitle ("Formulas and Equations for Spelling the Sounds of Spoken English") of her teaching manual, *Situation Spelling* (Cox 1977). The term "situation spelling" refers to the fact that the spelling of a particular speech sound tends to vary with its position in a particular word. In this manual, Cox states

> By studying systematically each sound and its most likely symbols in every significant position in monosyllabic and multisyllabic words, the student can eventually incorporate all of his knowledge of spelling the separate sounds in base words into his reflexes. (Cox 1977)

Cox's remedial program, which has reportedly been successful with dyslexic children and adults in tutoring, clinical, and small class settings, presents a challenge to instructors as well as students because of its level of sophistication. Multisensory techniques are incorporated into teaching at all levels of the program, as in the Orton-Gillingham system, and spelling practice uses the *simultaneous oral spelling (SOS)* method.

Sister Marie Grant has developed an instructional program for at-risk first grade students, using what she calls a *kinesthetic approach* (Grant 1985). These children are taught handwriting and spelling before reading. As soon as letter formations are stable, the children begin spelling practice via a linguistic approach that applies the principle of minimal contrasts. They are presented with c-v-c words differing only in initial consonants (for example, "hat," "bat," "mat") and are encouraged to discriminate and distinguish specific letter features spontaneously. The importance of letter sequencing is stressed by using the same group of letters to make different words (for example, "pan," "nap," "ten," "net"), in a simplified version of Cox's situation spelling. Following the principles of Johnson and My-

SHORT VOWEL SOUNDS

(ă) Voiced

I. REGULAR FOR SPELLING   Example

  A. Initial or Medial Position in a Base Word

      (ă) = a (in a closed syllable)   apple*

  B. Final Position in a Base Word - never in English words.

  ┌───┐
  │ Formula: Application: │
  │   │
  │ Sound Situation = Symbol   Pronunciation = Spelling   │
  │ 1⁺syl b.w._(ă)c = 1⁺syl b.w._ac   (ă'p'l) = apple   │
  └───┘

  Etymology: The letter a is never doubled in English words.

  Pronunciation: The speech sound (ă) is in the middle of the scale in
                     tone. The production opens the speaker's mouth wider
                     than does (ĕ) and less wide than (ŏ). The student can
                     associate tone, mouth shape, and kinesthetic memory for
                     spelling reinforcement if he practices while watching
                     his own mouth in a small mirror.

II. IRREGULAR FOR SPELLING (rare):   Example

  A. Initial or Medial Position in a Base Word

      (ă) = au (in a very few words)   laugh

  B. Final Position in a Base Word - never in English words.

  ┌───┐
  │ Formula: Application: │
  │ 1⁺syl b.w._(ă) = 1⁺syl b.w._au   (lăf) = laugh ˎ   │
  └───┘

                        Learned Words

              au   Misc.
              laugh   plait
              aunt   morale
              etc.

A Lesson from Situation Spelling by Aylett R. Cox. (Reproduced with permission from Educators Publishing Service, Inc., Cambridge, MA. Copyright 1977.)

klebust (1967), Grant separates phonetically spelled words from inconsistently spelled or nonphonetic words.

The unique aspect of Grant's remedial approach is the introduction of *hand motions to represent letter sounds*. The procedure for spelling the word "be," for instance, involves the student's learning the hand motions for long /e/ and for /b/, pronouncing the letter sounds and then blending the letter sounds before writing the word on the chalkboard. Grant contends that working initially at the chalkboard allows "for more muscular perception." After writing the word successfully on the chalkboard, the student practices writing the word on paper.

Grant has provided empirical support for this approach by comparing its effect over a four-year period on spelling, as well as reading, to a traditional approach which taught reading before writing and spelling. Sub-jects in the control group, taught by traditional methods, though not determined to be at-risk, were matched for IQ with subjects in the experimental group. By fourth grade, testing indicated that the mean spelling ability of experimental subjects was markedly superior to that of the control subjects. This finding, however, fails to indicate which aspects of the experimental treatment—the kinesthetic input, the sequencing of learning tasks, or some other instructional variable—was most responsible for the gains.

In their program, *Auditory Discrimination in Depth (A.D.D.)*, Charles and Pat Lindamood emphasize that, in order to spell, contrasts in spoken language must be perceived before contrasts in written language can be understood (Lindamood and Lindamood 1975). They maintain that many children do not naturally acquire the degree of phonological knowledge, or auditory-perceptual skills, needed for proficient spelling or reading. After working for many years with dyslexic individuals, Lindamood and Lindamood conclude:

> The one factor common to all of these students was their lack of auditory-perceptual skill, with its attendant problem in self-monitoring their production of specific sounds and sequences while pronouncing words, or monitoring and integrating sound-symbol identities and sequences during reading and spelling activities. (Lindamood and Lindamood 1975, Book 1)

Spelling instruction in the Lindamood program begins essentially with auditory conceptualization. A distinctive and important feature of this program is the attention brought to bear on sound production and the labeling of all letter sounds according to the oral movements involved in articulating these sounds. The sounds /b/ and /p/, for example, are called "lip poppers"; /f/ and /v/ are called "lip coolers." The student is taught to discriminate sounds in nonsense words by manipulating cards with pictures representing these sound labels. She then progresses to working with colored blocks that represent the sounds (the colors have no specific relationship to the letters but serve only to differentiate one sound from another). Once she can perform this task proficiently with single syllables, the student is given letter symbols to manipulate in spelling activities. Spelling instruction progresses from single to multisyllable words, starting in each case with nonsense words and moving to real words.

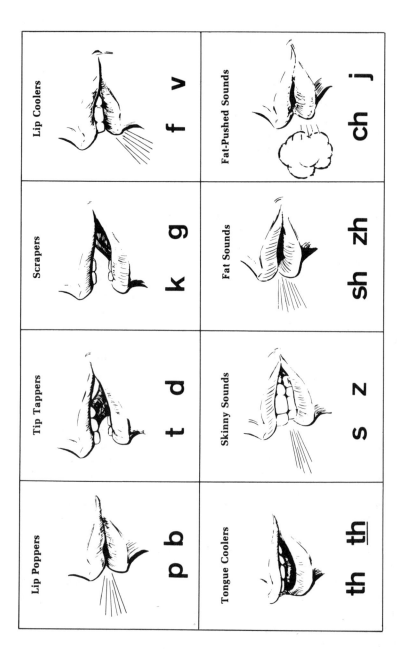

Letter Sound Labels. The A.D.D. Program: Auditory Discrimination in Depth by *Charles H. Lindamood and Patricia C. Lindamood. (Reproduced with permission from DLM Teaching Resources, Allen, TX. Copyright 1975.)*

Chapter 13 describes the Lindamood and Lindamood program in greater detail, as well as the Slingerland and Alphabetic Phonics programs, and cites the research to date on their success in teaching both spelling and reading to dyslexic students. Although we have substantial evidence that these and other instructional programs do work with dyslexic students, we need to determine which aspects of these programs are the most influential and why. Specifically, we need to know the value of multisensory procedures, to determine if, how, and why they help dyslexic students learn to spell.

CHAPTER

Handwriting Instruction

Beatrice Furner characterizes handwriting development as a perceptual learning process in which the learner must actively participate in order to internalize the procedures for letter formations (Furner 1983). An important aspect of perceptual learning is the ability to discriminate characteristic features. She criticizes most existing instructional programs for placing too much emphasis on tracing and copying procedures and not enough on active learning. Although there is a place for these procedures in early writing instruction, in and of themselves they do not force children to discriminate between letter shapes and to note the distinguishing characteristics of each letter.

When compared with tracing, copying seems to promote better learning (Askov and Greff 1975; Hirsch and Niedermeyer 1973); the explanation has been that copying involves a greater degree of visualization and attention to detail (Askov and Greff 1975). Joanna Williams (1975) has found that both copying and letter discrimination training contribute to handwriting development but in different ways: discrimination training, as in a matching-to-sample procedure, tends to generalize to new letters, whereas copying does not (each letter has to be learned individually). However, when compared to demonstration of letter formations or verbal description of rules for these formations or a combination of these two techniques, copying is found to be the least effective technique (Kirk 1981). C. Jan and Joan Wright designed flip-books, one for each lower-case letter which they gave to first-graders to use during independent practice (Wright and Wright 1980). When the children flip the books, the letter formations appear much as in animated cartoons. This innovative method has proved more successful than copying from static models; not only do the flip-books serve to demonstrate formational procedures, but the children enjoy using them, which adds a motivational factor.

Furner maintains that both discrimination and production are important processes in handwriting development, though they are useful for different reasons, and urges that demonstration and verbalization of letter formations replace the copying and tracing that predominates in handwriting instruction. In her own work, Furner combines perceptual learning principles with problem-solving methods, using questioning and discovery techniques, and she reports data supporting this approach (see Furner 1983 for a list of these principles). Although her research, as well as the research she reviews, deals with normal kindergarten and first-grade children, there is no reason to believe that it should not apply to dyslexic learners.

Regina Cicci, in addressing the writing problems of dyslexic students, lists seven forms of handwriting difficulties that may accompany dyslexia: incorrect pencil grasp, excessive tension in pencil grasp, incorrect position of paper, inappropriate size and spacing of letters and words, poor visual memory for letter formations, slow rate, and poor fine motor coordination, or dysgraphia. She suggests compensatory modifications to help dyslexic children and adolescents cope in the regular classroom; such modifications include using parents as scribes and proof readers, accepting taped or oral reports, and reducing length of written assignments (see Cicci 1983 for a complete list).

The question of how far to go in making allowances for poor handwriting in the classroom is an age-old dilemma. As teachers of dyslexic students, we must be aware of and sensitive to the difficulty they experience with written assignments and the added frustration that a handwriting problem can create. At the same time, we must try to prepare these students for the challenges that lie ahead when they may not be afforded compensatory support. One of the strongest arguments for devoting considerable time and energy to handwriting instruction with dyslexic students is that handwriting provides kinesthetic and visual reinforcement of spelling knowledge.

Many of the instructional principles advocated by Furner may be found in remedial handwriting programs for dyslexic children, most particularly those programs based on the Orton-Gillingham approach. For example, Alphabetic Phonics (Cox 1984) and Slingerland (1971) incorporate teacher demonstration, combined with verbal directions for particular letter strokes which the student repeats while forming the letters. *The Johnson Handwriting Program* (Johnson 1977), which Cox advocates for her

Perceptual Patterns Desk Card, The Johnson Handwriting Program. *(Reproduced with permission from Educators Publishing Service, Inc., Cambridge, MA. Copyright 1977.)*

students once they have received training in cursive writing in her program, teaches three *control strokes* as the basis of all cursive letter formations: the "drop stroke," the "anchor turn" (made directly on the base line), and the "release stroke." Cox adds a fourth classification, the "approach stroke" which she breaks down into four subcategories—"swing-under-up-stop,"—for the first approach stroke.

The Cox and Slingerland programs, as well as that of Diana King (1985), which is designed specifically to teach writing skills to adolescents, all require extensive tracing and copying. However, the inclusion of such practice is not arbitrary, as Furner implied it may be in some classrooms, but rather is considered an essential component of the multisensory training espoused by the authors of these programs. Other multisensory activities include King's prewriting exercises, such as "the windshield wiper" and "the wind tunnel," a series of circular scribbles that are done with eyes closed to develop rhythm, relaxation, and comfort in the handwriting situation, and Cox and Slingerland's *sky writing* which requires whole arm movements involving the gross-motor system.

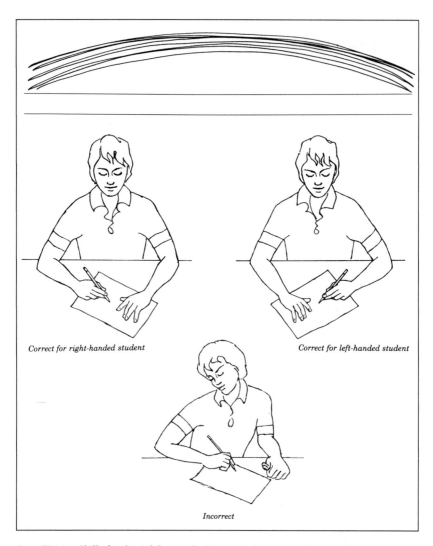

Correct for right-handed student   Correct for left-handed student

Incorrect

From Writing Skills for the Adolescent *by Diana Hanbury King. (Reproduced with permission from Educators Publishing Service, Inc., Cambridge, MA. Copyright 1985.)*

Correct sitting posture and *paper position* are stressed in these programs, the latter differing for left- and right-handed students. Left-handers are not allowed to hook their wrists in writing. Cox (1984) claims that handwriting retraining for dyslexic students who are not identified early is more difficult and time consuming than reading remediation. King (1985), who works mainly with adolescents, states, however, that true dysgraphia is extremely rare, despite the fact that the diagnosis is frequently made. She maintains that it is always worth the effort to develop good handwriting, and further, that with intensive retraining older students often make remarkable progress in a relatively short period of time. King and Cox both urge that dyslexic students learn to type, in addition to, but not in lieu of, developing handwriting skills.

King has in fact written an instructional manual called *Keyboarding Skills* (King 1986) to teach typing to dyslexic students in any grade. She describes her method as teaching "an alphabetic sequence with simultaneous oral spelling." The student learns by saying each letter aloud while typing it, which King believes establishes a conditioned reflex. She claims that many students can master the entire alphabet in less than an hour.

Whether to teach manuscript or cursive writing initially to dyslexic children has been a controversial issue over the years. Cox (1984) and King (1985) insist that cursive writing be used exclusively by dyslexic students. According to Cox, cursive writing reinforces left-right directionality, reduces reversals because the pencil is not raised off the paper, promotes rhythm and flow in letter formation, and eliminates the need to learn two writing systems. Furthermore, she contends, cursive letters are unique letter shapes and not mirror images of other letters. Beth Slingerland (1971) and Romalda Spalding (Spalding and Spalding 1986), on the other hand, advocate manuscript writing in order to conform to general school practices, as well as to avoid confusion with the type face in the child's readers. Cursive writing, in their programs, is not introduced until late second or third grade. There are truths in both positions which we teachers and clinicians should weigh before deciding which form of writing to teach our students. Student age will of course be an influential factor.

CHAPTER

Composition Instruction

Donald Graves, a leading authority on teaching writing, contended in 1978 that instruction in expressive writing is given short shrift in the education of American children. With dyslexic children, I must add, writing instruction has received even greater neglect, particularly at the elementary level. Although assessment of written language commands some attention in the learning disabilities literature (which includes dyslexia), remedial writing instruction is almost completely overlooked in methods textbooks for teachers of learning disabled students (Silverman et al. 1981). An investigation of eleven classrooms for learning disabled students reveals that less than one-tenth of the entire school day involved any writing activity on the part of students and, further, that seventy-five percent of that small fraction of time was spent copying (Leinhardt, Zigmond, and Cooley 1980). Among beginning readers, less than five minutes per day was spent producing written language, most of which consisted of single word responses to worksheet questions. Among students reading at second through fourth-grade levels, only 7.5 minutes of any school day was devoted to creative writing tasks.

According to Rita Silverman and her associates, some blame for the lack of written expression instruction in learning disabilities classrooms should be placed on teachers who have had limited writing experience themselves and have not been adequately trained to teach writing (Silverman et al. 1981). On the other hand, Edna Barenbaum (1983) points out that the omission of composition instruction with dyslexic and other language disabled children has been largely intentional, deriving from Helmer Myklebust's theory of language development (Myklebust 1965). Myklebust hypothesized that language abilities follow a hierarchical progression from Oral Receptive (listening) to Oral Expressive (speaking) to Written Receptive (reading) to Written Expressive (writing); in his view, a child is not ready to write until able to read. Thus, dyslexic students frequently do not receive instruction in written expression because their reading acquisition is delayed. If dyslexic students do receive writing instruction in the later elementary grades, the major emphasis is usually on grammar and mechanics (Barenbaum 1983).

A second theoretical vein of influence that has supported delaying composition instruction for dyslexic children is that of Samuel Orton (1937) and his associates, Anna Gillingham and Bessie Stillman (1960) who believed that spelling and mechanical difficulties constituted the major portion of the writing disabilities among these children. Fearing that free writing would only reinforce these problems, they advocated that children dictate their thoughts to tutors and not begin formal writing practice until high school. Orton and his colleagues did not concern themselves much with the plight of the dyslexic child in school; most of their suggestions were geared to clinical practice.

George Hillocks at the University of Chicago conducted a meta-analysis of the research related to teaching composition and determined that there are essentially four instructional modes: the presentational mode, the natural process mode, the environmental mode, and the individualized mode (Hillocks 1984). The *presentational mode,* also referred to as the *skills approach,* is by far the most common method used to teach written expression and is characterized by the teacher's playing the dominant role as the presenter of knowledge. In this approach, teaching objectives are clearly stated, information is provided in lectures or teacher-led discussions, samples of various writing styles are presented as models, specific assignments are given to students, and most of the feedback on student performance is provided by the teacher.

In sharp contrast to the skills approach, the *natural process mode* (Graves 1978) is characterized by the teacher's acting as "facilitator," whose primary role, as Hillocks describes it, is "to free the student's imagination and promote growth by sustaining a positive classroom atmosphere" (Hillocks 1984). Skill objectives in this approach are very general; the emphasis is placed on the student's writing about something that particularly interests him; the student shares his writing with his peers and receives feedback from them; editing, revision, and rewriting are strongly encouraged. The student exposed to this method learns by doing, rather than by studying principles or copying stylistic models. While the teacher exerts a subtle influence throughout the process in one-to-one conferences, the measure of success for a student's writing product is its reception by his peer critics.

The *environmental mode* combines aspects of both the presentational and process models and in many ways appears a compromise between the two. The objectives in this approach are clear and specific, the problems and assignments are selected by the teacher, and activities are structured by the teacher to be conducted by students initially in small groups and then followed through or replicated on an individual basis. This approach differs from the presentational mode, according to Hillocks, in that the principles and skills to be taught are not simply announced and illustrated but are taught by having students work through concrete problems. For example, if the skills goal was to enhance awareness of the writer's audience and to write for audience understanding, the assignment in the environmental model might be for each student to describe one of thirty types of shells so that other students would be able to select that particular shell from among the rest. Although each student creates his own individualized piece of writing, all students work on the same general topic or problem. The teacher helps the students establish the criteria for their writing through brief discussion of a sample of student writing. She acts as a guide for the group or for individual students only as long as needed, her major goal being to develop self-supporting behaviors in her students. Hillocks called this the "environmental" mode because it "brings teacher, student, and materials more nearly into balance and, in effect, takes advantage of all resources of the classroom." It might also be called the "interactive" mode.

The major distinction of the *individualized mode,* which Hillocks identifies in his meta-analysis of compositional instruction, is exactly as its label implies: one-to-one, or tutorial, instruction. Because he found it so variable, Hillocks does not describe this approach in any detail. However, he indicates that it tends to comprise aspects of either the environmental or presentational rather than the natural process approach.

The most important finding in Hillock's study is that the environmental mode is nearly three times as effective as either the presentational, natural process, or individualized mode of instruction. Furthermore, the most widely used approach, the presentational or skills model, was found to be the least effective. Additional outcomes worth noting are: (1) the study of grammar, as traditionally presented, does not improve, and in some instances even lowers, the quality of writing; (2) free writing is more effective than grammar instruction for enhancing writing quality, but less so than any other instructional focus; (3) sentence combining, or the practice of building more complex sentences from simpler ones, has a positive effect on the quality of written expression; (4) establishing criteria for students to become writing critics has a strong positive effect on written products; and (5) a problem solving approach, which Hillocks calls "inquiry," where students are presented with sets of information and asked to take a position or develop an argument, has an extremely positive effect on writing quality.

Despite the limited amount of research on teaching compositional skills to dyslexic children, the literature reveals a number of instructional principles and procedures that seem to be important. The first among them is the need to begin this instruction early, rather than waiting for reading or spelling skills to reach a particular level (Barenbaum 1983; Silverman et al. 1981). The importance of an optimal teaching environment has also been stressed. Donald Graves maintains that the classroom setting during writing instruction periods should be structured and highly predictable in terms of the time and frequency of occurrence and the consistency of teacher behavior. Writing instruction should take place at least four times a week and at set times, according to Graves. The teacher should create a "studio atmosphere," interacting with individual students as she moves around the room and letting them know that she is there to offer suggestions but not to solve their writing problems. Barenbaum emphasizes the need for a "safe" environment, by which she means one that is positive and reinforcing.

A major hurdle in working with dyslexic children is simply getting them to write. Asking them to keep journals from which they can later select writing topics, as Graves has suggested, may be requiring too much of these children, who have so many writing problems. Instead, nonthreatening prewriting activities, such as group discussion about topics of interest to the students, should provide motivation for written expression. Barenbaum makes a point of contrasting this practice with the group-dictated language experience approach, which she claims discourages individual initiative. However, it may be necessary to begin with the latter approach, as teachers of the Slingerland method tend to do, until students have gained enough confidence to work independently. Silverman and her colleagues recommend that during this period the teacher and students generate questions that become the framework for students' creative writing. For younger dyslexic students who are just beginning to write, Barenbaum proposes having them label pictures or conduct short word counts. For reluctant adolescent writers, Diana King (1985) suggests providing lists of words with which to construct single sentences.

The establishment of an audience for writing activities is another important component of successful writing instruction. Graves strongly advocates *peer sharing* and *peer feedback*. Barenbaum urges that students' writing be displayed in the classroom and school library in book form, as well as in other ways. In my own practice, as well as in classroom observations, I have found that having students illustrate and bind their own written work in book form can be a tremendously rewarding experience.

Teacher-student conferences are core activities in both the process and environmental models of writing instruction, not only for encouragement and guidance, but for developing the practice of drafting and revising (Barenbaum 1983; Graves 1985; Silverman et al. 1981). The early emphasis in these conferences is on meaning. Not until the student reaches a certain level of fluency is attention paid to mechanics and spelling, and then only in small and judiously applied doses. Even Diana King, who adheres to a skills approach, cautioned against discouraging students by focusing on errors. In her program, tutors are prohibited from placing red marks on student papers for at least a year after remediation has begun and are advised never to correct all errors on a page (King 1985). Donald Graves makes several suggestions about error corrections in teacher-student conferences: (1) identify and remediate errors in order of importance; (2) choose only one particular error to correct at a given time; (3) focus on specific writing problems as the need arises; (4) provide more than one experience to remediate the problem (Graves 1983).

Edna Barenbaum adds two activities for teachers to undertake that contribute to enhancing the written expression of dyslexic children (Barenbaum 1983). One is *keeping careful records of student writing activities.* An appealing suggestion made by Graves (1983) for this purpose is to have each student keep a folder to contain his work and have the student and teacher use the four sides of the folder to record relevent information on the student's progress; this might include, for example, the pieces of writing he has done, the skills he has learned, topics about which he may want to write. A second activity is to provide a *broad language base,* through oral language activities and through exposure to literature.

Diana King's writing program, *Writing Skills for the Adolescent* (1985), is based on Orton-Gillingham principles and is intended to interface with Orton-Gillingham reading instruction. This is probably the most comprehensive writing program developed to date for dyslexic students since it deals with handwriting, spelling, and formulation. It is designed essentially as a tutorial program for college-bound adolescent dyslexic boys, many of whom are diagnosed late. King's approach is exceedingly pragmatic, most probably because time is of the essence with these students. Her program involves extensive retraining in handwriting, as well as remediation of spelling, mechanical, and formulational difficulties. Attitudinal problems must also be dealt with, as most students have experienced many years of failure, and King takes the position that any form of confidence building, even if it requires writing simple sentences with lists of words, justifies the tedium of a particular task.

In King's program, writing instruction begins in conjunction with spelling instruction, by having students compose simple sentences from lists of spelling words. Once this activity can be accomplished with some facility, formal grammar instruction begins. In her manual for tutors, King points out that grammar is important for college-bound students;

she tells these students they can learn all they need to know in just a few months. Grammar study begins with parts of speech, moves on to the study of various types of clauses, and ends with what King calls "verbals": participles, gerunds, and infinitives. King maintains that grammar is best taught by having students write single sentences (simple, compound, and complex), rather than relying on workbook exercises.

The student in King's writing program progresses from sentences to paragraphs to essays. King places considerable emphasis on paragraph construction which she views as "an exercise in logical thinking." Instruction begins with the generation of a list of words to provide topics for paragraph writing, then the production of several statements to support a topic sentence, then the composition of a topic sentence, and finally the weaving together of all the sentences. Students are taught to distinguish and to write various types of paragraphs, for example, the *definition paragraph,* the *narrative paragraph,* or the *process paragraph* which describes some procedure. Instruction in essay writing follows the same pattern as paragraph writing. The student is taught to provide an introductory paragraph that includes a thesis statement, followed by several supporting paragraphs, each having a topic sentence, and ending with a concluding paragraph. King's basic essay model contains five paragraphs.

Although she has no quantitative data to confirm the effectiveness of her program, in the appendix of her teaching manual King includes before-and-after writing samples from some of her students. She has written a brief educational history for each case, which, combined with the writing samples, provides substantial support for her program. She places the major instructional emphasis on expository writing, probably because it is a critical priority for the college-bound adolescent, and gives little attention to creative writing, at least in her instruction manual.

The use of *word processing programs* for writing instruction is in its early stages; however, there is a small body of research that has investigated its use with learning disabled students, many of whom we can assume are dyslexic. Some of the observed advantages of computerized word processing for these students include: the ability to produce a neat, easy-to-read, printed copy which provides the student with feedback on his writing and may also increase his motivation; the ability to edit and revise without tedious recopying; and the ability to type, which can compensate for poor handwriting (MacArthur and Schneiderman 1986). A major advantage from the teacher's standpoint is that the computer provides a picture of the student's writing process. It also allows her to interact with the student in collaborative writing activities which can be extremely facilitative toward improving the quality and quantity of the student's writing (Morocco and Neuman 1986).

At the same time, these factors may not always be advantages. Studies have identified several potentially negative aspects of word processing with learning disabled students. Typing, for example, has been found in some cases to be an obstacle, and slow speed may eliminate any advantages of word processing. In a recent study with fifth- and sixth-grade learning disabled students, word processing proved to be less than half as fast as handwriting (MacArthur and Graham 1988). Learning and remembering the editing commands, knowing how to use spaces and returns and how to save and load information may also present roadblocks (MacArthur and Schneiderman 1986). Word processing may or may not lead to greater quantity of writing than does handwriting. Joyce Steeves contends that writing with a computer produces much longer pieces than writing with pencil and paper (Steeves 1987); Charles MacArthur and Ben Schneiderman also have found this to be true (MacArthur and Schneiderman 1986). In sharp contrast, a recent investigation with learning disabled fifth- and sixth-graders revealed no significant differences between handwriting and word processing in length or any other important dimension: "length, quality, story structure, mechanical or grammatical errors, vocabulary, or average T-unit length"[1] (MacArthur and Graves 1988). Furthermore, word processing may not lead to more spontaneous revision, although under teacher supervision students seem willing to revise (Mokros and Russell 1986). A nationwide survey on the use of computers with special needs students found that computers tended not to be used for drafts but only for final copies of written work (Mokros and Russell 1986). Charles MacArthur and Steve Graham recently found that instead of encouraging greater focus on content as opposed to mechanics on the first draft of a writing piece, word processing induced students to spend more time correcting minor errors (MacArthur and Graham 1988).

There appear to be two pivotal factors in the success of any word processing program with dyslexic students. The first is the competence of the teacher who must act in a supervisory position, since no program will be effective if students are left unsupervised. The teacher needs to be comfortable in using computers, knowledgeable about computer programs, and thoroughly familiar with the program she selects. Further, she needs to decide how interactive to be in the lessons she conducts and when not to intrude in a student's writing process. Too much teacher involvement can pose problems of control over the written product (Morocco and Neuman 1986).

The second factor is the mode of instruction for which the word processing program is being applied, whether it be a skills approach that focuses on mechanics or a process approach that stresses content and encourages revision; on its own, no word processing program will have a

---

[1] A T-unit is a segment of written language that has a subject and verb and therefore could stand on its own as a meaningful sentence.

significant effect on the writing of dyslexic students (MacArthur and Graham 1988). I believe there is a place for both these instructional approaches in working with dyslexic as well as normally achieving students.

At the moment, there is no word processing program deemed best for dyslexic students, and there is certainly not room enough here to mention the various programs currently available. However, as teachers, we will make better decisions in selecting appropriate word processing programs for our students if we educate ourselves in the use of computers, keep abreast of the research on new programming and bear in mind the critical factors that I have discussed.

CHAPTER

11

The Reading-Writing Relationship

The relationship between reading and writing has captured the attention of a number of respected theorists who believe that reading and writing are mutually facilitative skills. These theorists have questioned the standard classroom practice of delaying writing activities until reading skills have been acquired, and have advocated that, at the very least, reading and writing should be taught together.

Maria Montessori (1964) was perhaps the first educator to suggest that writing precedes reading developmentally and that it is thus more natural for children to begin reading instruction by composing their own words, rather than by attempting to read the words of others. One of the strongest proponents of Montessori's view has been Carol Chomsky (1979) who feels that when children start school they are better able to apply their own language to encode meaning than to decode meaning from formal printed language. Chomsky believes, as did Montessori, that building an awareness of the communicative purposes of written language is one of the primary advantages of having children write before teaching them to read. In addition, she maintains that this approach enhances phonological awareness. From her observations of children composing self-generated stories as part of their first grade schooling, Chomsky concluded:

> The invented spellers, during the months that they engage in their writing
> activities, are providing themselves with excellent and valuable practice in

phonetics, word analysis and synthesis, and letter-sound correspondences. (Chomsky 1979)

Uta Frith recently proposed a developmental model of reading acquisition that concurs with Chomsky's conclusions (Frith 1986). Paraphrasing Frith, Sylvia Farnham-Diggery cites the advantages of early writing activities: " . . . the writing process requires segmenting and sequencing and thus sets up the conditions for the discovery of the alphabetic principle." (Farnham-Diggery 1986a)

One of the major concerns raised about this approach is that it may perpetuate incorrect spellings. This is the position held by most Orton-Gillingham trained teachers who work with dyslexic children. As mentioned earlier (see page 110), these remedial educators do not introduce free writing activities until their pupils have mastered basic phonics skills, although copying and practice in writing from dictation forms a substantial portion of their curriculum. However, Chomsky, as well as Charles Read (1975) and Glenda Bissex (1980), in observations of kindergarten and first grade nondyslexic children, have found that invented spellings are gradually replaced with conventional spellings as the children gain reading experience. These investigators also noted remarkable consistency in the patterns of spelling approximations among the children. The letter *H,* for example, is frequently used to represent the digraph *ch.*

A second concern about the writing-before-reading approach to teaching is that children may be confused by the differences between their own spellings and the printed words they encounter when they begin to read. This too is not a problem, according to Chomsky (1979). Reporting on Read's observations (Read 1970), she claims that children appear to have no difficulty making the distinction between their spellings and conventional spellings and that they tend, in fact, to view writing and reading as completely separate tasks, a conclusion that Lynette Bradley and Peter Bryant (1979, 1985) also reach in their research.

Timothy Shanahan investigated the reading-writing relationship with second- and fifth-grade students, by applying multivariate analysis to scores attained on various reading and writing tasks (Shanahan 1984). He found that, despite a significant relationship between the two skill areas, the degree to which skill in writing influences skill in reading and vice versa is no more than forty percent. In a second analysis, Shanahan with Richard Lomax attempted to determine the directionality of the relationship by constructing three theoretical models (reading-to-writing, writing-to-reading, and an interactive model) to represent the flow of influence (Shanahan and Lomax 1985). Results of the analysis indicate that reading has a stronger facilitative influence on writing than the other way around, but that the relationship is best represented by the interactive model. Furthermore, within the interactive model, the interaction between writing and reading is more significant at the word level than at the passage level and appears stronger in second grade than in fifth grade. Similarly, Connie Juel and her colleagues find the relationship to be greater at the word level and stronger with younger (first-grade) than with older (second-grade) children (Juel, Griffeth, and Gough 1985). Shanahan and Lomax suggest that these findings reflect the fact that considerably greater amount of instructional time is devoted to reading than to writing in our schools.

In one of the few efforts to explore the effects of writing on reading with reading disabled children, Lee Dobson in 1985 took eight first-graders who had failed to learn to read by mid-year and provided them with daily half-hour free-writing sessions. The children were encouraged to draw pictures and then write stories to accompany them. The teacher acted only as facilitator, never correcting their spelling errors, and when help was requested, deferring to the other children for their input rather than immediately providing the answer. Although he collected no quantitative data, Dobson maintains that notable progress is made in both writing and reading ability as a result of this activity. Many of the misspellings eventually drop out, though admittedly after a longer period of time than might be expected for normally achieving children. An especially important treatment outcome, Dobson believes, is the improved motivation among these children who had earlier met with failure.

The Spalding Method is a beginning reading program for classroom use that starts with spelling and writing. It was developed by Romalda Spalding. A teacher's manual for the program, called *The Writing Road to Reading,* was published in 1957 and has been recently revised (Spalding and Spalding 1986) with an introduction by Sylvia Farnham-Diggery, a psychologist and professor at the University of Delaware. Farnham-Diggery, who also runs the Reading Study Center at the university, states that she has used the Spalding Method with remarkable success for both beginning and remedial instruction, though she acknowledges the need for further documentation of its effectiveness with disabled readers.

Romalda Spalding was trained in the Orton-Gillingham approach by Dr. Orton and then went on to develop a language arts program that could be used with a whole class. Thus, the Spalding Method incorporates many of the Orton-Gillingham principles, including an emphasis on integrating the various sensory modalities involved in learning to read. However, it differs from the earlier method in many respects, most particularly by teaching writing before reading and by introducing first the most commonly used English words, many of which are not phonetically regular. The Orton-Gillingham approach, as previously mentioned, focuses primarily on words that have phonetic spelling patterns and introduces any that do not as exception words.

The Spalding Method teaches the set of phoneme-letter units or phonograms selected by Anna Gillingham in developing the Orton-

Gillingham program: the twenty-six letters of the alphabet and forty-four combinations of two, three, or four letters that make a single sound (for example, *ai, igh, ough*). Students are first taught to spell and write fifty-four of these phonograms and are then taught to spell and write 150 of the 1,700 most frequently used words. Teachers follow a general lesson script that involves saying the word to be learned, asking how many syllables it has, asking what is the first sound, and having students write the letter as she writes it on the chalkboard. The procedure continues until the word has been written.

Students write all words in notebooks which they add to as they proceed through the program. These spelling books serve as their major reference source. Manuscript writing is taught, primarily so as not to confuse students when they encounter print, but instruction in cursive writing usually begins by the middle of second grade. Twenty-nine spelling rules are taught in the program; students write these in their books along with examples of application. In addition, students are taught a marking system to help them identify and remember phonogram spellings and pronunciations: phonograms are underlined and, for those having more than one sound, numbers are used to identify which sound a phonogram represents in a given word. Farnham-Diggery maintains in her introduction to the program manual that knowing the seventy phonograms and these twenty-nine rules enables anyone to spell eighty percent of all English words.

Reading in the Spalding Method begins after students have mastered 150 words, that is, they can spell them aloud, write them from dictation, and read them. Rather than using a basal program, students read trade books from the beginning; Spalding has provided a list of suggested books for five grade levels in the program manual appendix. According to Farnham-Diggery, reading in this method is never taught; children "simply pick up a book and start reading" (Farnham-Diggery 1986b). She adds that the Spalding Method exposes them early to good literature and furthermore, encourages them to write their own stories, plays, and poems.

Whether or not a writing-before-reading approach is an effective way to teach dyslexic children is a question that calls for further exploration. Having children write words that they may not have learned by sight draws their attention to the sounds in those words and thereby enhances phonemic awareness. Writing also gives children a feeling of empowerment and ownership over the words they learn, increasing their motivation to learn more. I believe strongly that writing should play an equal role to reading at the start of any language arts curriculum. The recently developed Writing to Read program (Martin and Freidberg 1986), which contains a word processing component aimed at promoting reading acquisition among kindergarteners and first graders, may be a step in this direction. John Henry Martin, the author of this program, maintains that no cases of dyslexia were observed among some 10,000 children receiving Writing to Read instruction. Unfortunately, he did not describe the learning characteristics of the three to five percent of these children who failed to respond to this instruction, except to say that they had extremely limited oral vocabularies.

PART III

Reading Programs for Dyslexic Students

The chapters that follow provide information on instructional programs that serve as alternatives to basal reader programs for teaching reading, writing, and spelling skills. Most of these programs were designed for children who are dyslexic or who might be at risk for reading failure. They include Alphabetic Phonics, the Slingerland Program, Recipe for Reading, Enfield and Greene's Project Read, the Lindamoods' Auditory Discrimination in Depth, DISTAR and Corrective Reading. Some of these programs can be considered remedial, others preventive or developmental; yet others are used for both purposes.

Although several of these programs derive from the Orton-Gillingham multisensory approach, each is unique in a number of important respects. The instructional settings for which they have been developed range from tutorials to whole classrooms. The breadth of their curricula varies from almost exclusive focus on decoding, spelling, and handwriting to the incorporation of reading comprehension and expressive writing skills. DISTAR, which was originally developed as a beginning reading program for culturally or economically disadvantaged children, is included here because of its subsequent use with children classified as learning disabled, many of whom might be considered dyslexic. Except for Corrective Reading, an extension of DISTAR designed for fourth- through twelfth-grade underachieving students, all of these programs are suited to children in the early elementary grades; most, however, are adaptable for older children and some even for adults.

Two additional programs are described that were not designed specifically for dyslexic or reading disabled children: Writing to Read and Calfee's Project READ. I have included them because they represent a significant departure from the traditional basal approach and incorporate many of the instructional principles and teaching methods that research has shown to be effective with dyslexic students.

Each program is described in terms of its basic rationale, or theoretical perspective, its curriculum and instructional methodology, its teacher training requirements, and, where information is available, its effectiveness. The descriptions should be taken as overviews rather than comprehensive investigations. I have not attempted to compare the programs or to single out the one "best" program. Instead, I hope that the information provided in the previous chapters on the nature of dyslexia and the instructional requirements of dyslexic students have afforded readers of this book a theoretical framework with which to make their own judgments on the relative value of any of these programs for students with whom they are concerned. The last chapter, Curriculum Planning for Dyslexic Students, discusses the major circumstantial factors that influence the delivery of effective reading and language arts instruction to these students.

CHAPTER 12

Alphabetic Phonics

BACKGROUND AND RATIONALE

Alphabetic Phonics is an adaptation of the Orton-Gillingham multi-sensory approach to teaching language arts to dyslexic children that has been designed for use in small group, as well as one-to-one tutorial settings. The program began in the mid 1960s at Scottish Rite Hospital in Dallas, Texas with the collaboration of Sally Childs (a colleague of Anna Gillingham), Lucius Waites (a neuro-pediatrician who established a remedial clinic at the hospital), and Aylett Cox (a teacher who wrote the Alphabetic Phonics curriculum). The curriculum was developed and revised over a ten-year period, during which over 1,000 dyslexic children came to Waite's clinic for remedial instruction. In order to meet the needs of all the children referred, teaching at Scottish Rite was expanded from tutorials to small groups.

Alphabetic Phonics is built upon Samuel Orton's theories about dyslexia and incorporates multisensory activities to provide linkages between the visual, auditory, and kinesthetic senses. To this theoretical framework, the program has added a discovery approach to learning. The term alphabetic phonics refers to "a structured system of teaching students the coding patterns of the English language" (Cox 1985). The program represents a reorganization, refinement, and elaboration of the Orton-Gillingham approach to teaching dyslexic children. Justification for these changes is based on several assumptions, the first being the aforementioned need to serve a greater number of children and to serve them, wherever possible, within traditional schools.

A second assumption, which is more vulnerable to question, is that up to 20 percent of any class entering elementary school will not respond to traditional classroom instruction. Aylett Cox maintains that the major problem of these dyslexic children is their inability to process two-dimensional linguistic symbols, despite the presence of often superior three-dimensional skills. She contends that most children who are not dyslexic develop "strong, reliable photographic memories for 2-dimensional symbols" (Cox 1983). An additional assumption offered in support of her adaptation of the Orton-Gillingham approach is that the majority (85 percent) of the 30,000 most commonly used English words can be considered phonetically regular and therefore predictable (Cox 1983).

CURRICULUM AND INSTRUCTION

The Alphabetic Phonics curriculum is highly structured and sequentially organized. It is extremely comprehensive in that it covers many aspects of language acquisition, including listening skills, and extends from very basic ability levels, such as letter recognition, to sophisticated levels of linguistic knowledge, such as syllabicating and coding polysyllabic words. As they progress through the curriculum, students are taught an extensive vocabulary to apply to their language learning, which includes technical terms such as "medial" (referring to letters or sounds occurring in the middle of words), "kinesthetic," "modality," and "morpheme." Judith Birsh, an Alphabetic Phonics teacher trainer, refers to this terminology as a "meta-language," a language with which to talk about language (Birsh 1988). Students are also taught a set of code marks that indicate the speech sounds of each letter or combination of letters and a lengthy list of symbols and abbreviations related to word decoding, for example "d.m." for diacritical mark, "2 + syl b.w." for a base word of two or more syllables. In addition, they learn a set of six formulas for spelling words and a set of four formulas for syllable division.

The curriculum is too complex to describe here in detail; it is outlined in a master guide for teachers, *Structures and Techniques* (Cox 1984), as well as in two companion books, *Situation Reading* and *Situation Spelling,* all available through Educators Publishing Service. Instead, I will mention the program's major components and most distinguishing characteristics.

Twelve primary instructional principles or techniques are applied in the Alphabetic Phonics curriculum (Cox 1983):

1. Focus on essential processes, not products.
2. Provide enough practice to ensure mastery and automaticity.

3. Organize instruction within general daily master lesson plans.
4. Change activities often.
5. Teach from the known (oral language) to the unknown (written language).
6. Lead students to discover prevailing concepts through Socratic questioning.
7. Emphasize the law of probability.
8. Teach cursive handwriting.
9. Provide semantic clues and/or a rationale for any material that must be memorized.
10. Use criterion-referenced tests (Bench Mark Measures), not only to ensure mastery and measure progress, but also to inform students of their progress.
11. Teach all basic sound-symbol relationships and develop word attack skills.
12. Emphasize the importance of appropriate positions for all learning activities (reading, handwriting at desk and at chalkboard, etc.).

The structured daily lesson takes an hour to complete; the time spent on any activity ranges from 60 seconds to 10 minutes. A typical lesson contains the following activities (Cox 1985):

1. An alphabetic activity, which emphasizes sequence and directionality.
2. Introduction of a new element or concept, which begins with discovery and is reinforced with multisensory techniques.
3. Training in automatic recognition of letter names, through flashcard presentation (Reading Decks).
4. Training in recognition of letter sounds, by having students pronounce the sounds for a letter or letters presented on flashcards (Spelling Decks) and then naming and writing the letter or letters.
5. Practice in reading and spelling (10 minutes allotted for each). Each task is continued until student reaches 95 percent mastery, as measured by the Bench Mark Measures.
6. Handwriting practice.
7. Practice in verbal expression, first oral and later written, focusing on various skills (e.g., sequencing ideas, creative expression, vocabulary, syntax).
8. Listening to good literature and building comprehension skills, while reading instruction focuses on decoding skills.

Throughout instruction, auditory, visual, and kinesthetic channels are linked in all possible ways. Spelling is reinforced, for example, with sky-writing. Cursive handwriting is taught from the beginning, the rationale being that it encourages left-right directionality, as well as sound blending, and considerable emphasis is placed on teaching cursive letter formations. As mentioned in Chapter 9, four basic control strokes are taught (see pp. 104–105). A discovery, or learning through experience, approach via one or more of the sensory channels is used to introduce new concepts. For instance, for teaching the concept of vowels, students are told to say aloud short *a* (/ăăăă/) and then asked a series of questions which will lead them to discover the various properties of vowels: "What are you doing with your mouth? Is it open or closed?"; "Put your hand on your throat. What do you feel?" The teacher then supplies the appropriate terms for their answers; students learn that vowels are open and voiced sounds.

Lessons in the early stages begin with a five minute teacher presentation on the development of language. Each lesson also includes a review of new elements introduced that day. Most of the materials used have been designed for the program or are teacher-made, though the linguistic reading series, *Let's Read* (Bloomfield, Barnhart, and Barnhart 1965), is used for reading practice.

As its name implies, Alphabetic Phonics stresses the unique characteristics of the English alphabet, most particularly phonology and letter sequence, and places major emphasis on teaching phonic skills for reading and spelling. The term "situation learning" is applied to both reading and spelling and refers to the fact that the spelling of a letter sound may vary with its position in any word (see pp. 97–98). Thus the assumption of regularity or predictability of English spelling is maintained, but the demands placed on the student are substantial. He or she must learn to be a scientific speller. In Cox's words:

> By studying systematically each sound and its most likely symbols in every significant position in monosyllabic and multisyllabic words, the student can eventually incorporate all of this knowledge of spelling the separate sounds in base words into his reflexes. (Cox 1977)

Irregular spellings are presented as "learned words" that must be memorized.

According to Cox, 400 to 600 hours of multisensory instruction are required for dyslexic children to develop accuracy and automaticity in decoding and encoding. Reading comprehension instruction does not begin until decoding skills have reached a minimal level of accuracy and automaticity. Children remain in the program for at least two, and usually three, years. Completion of the highest level of programmed instruction, with 95 percent mastery on the Bench Mark Measures, ensures a minimum of seventh grade literacy (Roy 1986).

Practice in written expression is often initiated by having students create scrapbooks and then by encouraging them to keep logs. Composition usually begins as a group effort; independent writing is not undertaken until handwriting and spelling skills are reasonably developed (late second or early third year). Cox (1984) emphasizes the need for explicit instruction in grammar and syntax for dyslexic students as they move into expository writing. She suggests sentence diagramming for demonstration and practice. She also stresses the importance of helping these children to expand their word knowledge, but advocates teaching a few basic Greek and Latin roots and the most common prefixes and suffixes rather than lists of words. She maintains, as well, that dyslexic children will learn and retain new vocabulary more readily when guided to do so within experiential contexts, such as field trips, instead of through rote memory activities.

TEACHER TRAINING

Presently, there are at least five Alphabetic Phonics teacher training centers in the United States. They are located at: The Aylett Royall Cox Institute in Dallas, Texas; Scottish Rite Hospital in Lubbock, Texas; The Neuhaus Education Center in Houston, Texas; the Katheryne B. Paine Foundation in Oklahoma City, Oklahoma; and Teachers College, Columbia University, in New York City.

Training for teachers of Alphabetic Phonics is extensive (480 hours) and demanding. Teachers are required to attend a four-week introductory summer workshop and a two-week advanced workshop the following summer. These daily workshops last seven hours and include lectures, demonstrations, and practice. In addition, substantial reading and take-home projects are assigned. Trainees are required to teach the curriculum to individuals and small groups and are frequently observed and evaluated by support staff. They are not officially certified as Alphabetic Phonics teachers until the two-year training program is completed. The training is based on the need to fill three gaps in teacher education today: (1) knowledge of the structure of the English language; (2) knowledge of the science of phonetic spelling; and (3) a carefully structured curriculum, arranged in order of difficulty.

EVALUATION AND IMPLEMENTATION

Several evaluation studies of Alphabetic Phonics instruction have been conducted in the 1980s. Betty Roy (1986) investigated the effects of this training, administered in a clinic setting to a relatively small group of subjects, ages eight to fifteen, who were reading two to four years below grade level. Group mean gains on the Woodcock Reading Mastery Test showed greatest improvement in word attack and least in word recogni-

since phonetic analysis is a primary focus of the curriculum. Spelling progress, assessed by the Bench Mark Measures, lagged behind reading. Although Roy does not present individual achievement gains, she states that there was considerable variation in levels of improvement between subjects.

The major problem with all the Alphabetic Phonics studies reported to date, including Roy's, is the lack of control groups. Mikel Brightman (1986) reports significant improvement in spelling, as measured by a standardized test, for first through third grade students in one school who were enrolled in Alphabetic Phonics; this finding applies to both predictable and unpredictable spellings; but since the study did not include a comparison group of dyslexic students who did not receive Alphabetic Phonics training, it cannot be claimed without reservation that the training itself was responsible for the improvement.

Ronald Frankiewicz (1985) used the individual change model of research design to evaluate the effectiveness of the Alphabetic Phonics curriculum with thirteen students receiving one-to-one instruction over a period of 170 to 190 hours. In this study each subject provided his own baseline; the variability of his gain scores among various subskills was taken into account in estimating his overall reading improvement. According to Frankiewicz, though time consuming, this method is more sensitive to the effects of individually administered instruction than the group comparison approach. He maintains that summaries of each individual's progress can be used to describe a program's overall impact. Results of this study indicate an average growth rate of nearly 60 percent across all Woodcock Reading Mastery subtests.

An earlier study (Frankiewicz 1984) examined growth trends in various skill areas over several years for sixth-, seventh-, and eighth-grade students taught Alphabetic Phonics in small group settings. The study yielded some interesting differences in growth rate patterns among reading subskills—periods of rapid acceleration, for example, and periods of leveling off—which would seem to be valuable information for curriculum developers. Frankiewicz maintains that the dyslexic subjects in all three grades made greater improvement in most skill areas than would be expected of normal children within the same amount of time. He does not indicate, however, his data source for determining expected growth rate for normal children. In the absence of a true control group, Frankiewicz's data do not prove Alphabetic Phonics more effective than another remedial approach, though they do demonstrate academic progress for dyslexic children receiving Alphabetic Phonics training.

Whether or not Alphabetic Phonics is cost effective is an important question, particularly in view of its intensive teacher training requirements and the fact that the program usually serves as an addition, rather than as a replacement for the traditional language arts curriculum. The question can best be answered by comparing Alphabetic Phonics with other intervention approaches to the problems of dyslexia.

ADAPTATIONS OF ALPHABETIC PHONICS

Margaret Smith and Edith Hogan, both former Alphabetic Phonics teacher trainers, have revised the Alphabetic Phonics curriculum for whole classroom use. They call their program the Multisensory Teaching Approach (MTA). Smith and Hogan maintain that the MTA program can be incorporated into other reading programs in regular classrooms, or used as a remedial program with dyslexic students.

Training for teaching the MTA program involves a two-week, day-long basic course, which includes lectures, daily practicum, and observations. This training is offered by Edmar Educational Services in Dallas, Texas. Training to become an academic language therapist, which is also offered by Edmar, requires taking the basic two-week course, plus two years of practicum during the school year, four advanced workshops and six individual consultation/demonstrations scheduled periodically during the two-year period, and an additional two weeks of instruction.

Smith and Hogan have recently developed a kit that contains the essential instruction manuals and materials needed for teaching the program. The manuals provide more specific instruction for teachers than do the original Alphabetic Phonics manuals, including lesson scripts. The MTA kit is distributed by Educators Publishing Service in Cambridge, Massachusetts. Several Alphabetic Phonics specialists have informed me that the kit is an excellent resource for any Alphabetic Phonics teacher.

A four-year evaluation study of MTA instruction was conducted in Texas, where it was implemented in a public school in both remedial and nonremedial classes (Vickery, Reynolds, and Cochran 1987). Scores on the California Achievement Test (CAT) indicated that children in grades three, five, and six who had received MTA instruction made, on average, significantly greater progress in reading and spelling than children in the same classes in previous years who did not receive this instruction. The amount of gain tended to increase with the number of years of exposure to MTA instruction. Fourth-grade children, however, did not evidence this advantage. Further research on the effectiveness of MTA is underway.

Another adaptation of the Alphabetic Phonics curriculum has recently been developed by Lucius Waites and Anna Ramey at Scottish Rite Hospital in Dallas, Texas. This is a two-year program, intended for dyslexic students or students considered to be at risk for dyslexia. Called the Dyslexia Training Program, the core of its curriculum is a cumulative series of 350 one-hour taped Alphabetic Phonics lessons. The major advantage of the program, according to its developers, is that it does not require the extensive teacher training of the original Alphabetics Phonics curriculum. The classroom teacher, referred to as a proctor, learns the program while it is in progress, from the video tapes and from the teacher's guides. These guides and student workbooks, as well as the Bloomfield–Barnhart's *Let's Read* books used in the program, are available from Educators Publishing Service, while the tapes must be ordered from the Texas Scottish Rite Hospital Dyslexia Program. At the present time (1988), video tapes have been made for only the first year of instruction.

It is too soon to ascertain the effectiveness of the Dyslexia Training Program. However, I question the assumption that the Alphabetic Phonics curriculum can be taught without prior teacher training in the curriculum. Furthermore, a certain amount of vitality is lost when the teacher directs lessons from a previously filmed tape rather than teaching the lessons to the class herself. In addition, the relatively high cost of the equipment needed for implementing the Dyslexia Training Program, in addition to the instruction materials required, must be considered.

CHAPTER

13

Auditory Discrimination in Depth

BACKGROUND AND RATIONALE

Auditory Discrimination in Depth (ADD) was developed by Charles and Patricia Lindamood, the former an English teacher, the latter a speech pathologist, as a preventive, developmental, or remedial program to teach auditory conceptualization skills basic to reading, spelling, and speech. The program is designed to complement any reading program. It can be used with kindergarten children to bolster the development of auditory–perceptual awareness, as well as with children and adults who fail to read and spell successfully because of failure to acquire phonemic analysis skills.

The Lindamoods (1980) draw attention to the importance of self-correction for language learning and literacy acquisition and to the fact that this skill requires auditory conceptualization judgment, which they define as "the ability to perceive the identity, number, and sequence of speech sounds in spoken patterns, and to perceive *how* and *where* patterns are different." As mentioned in Chapter 4 in the section entitled Training in Phonological Awareness, the Lindamood Auditory Conceptualization (LAC) test measures this ability. The Lindamoods claim to have found a surprising number of adults, involved in many professions (banking, engineering, medicine, teaching, etc.), with hidden deficits in this area. They have called these individuals "closet illiterates."

The Lindamoods have been able to demonstrate strong correlations between LAC scores and word recognition, reading comprehension, and spelling scores on various standardized tests. Their research led them to conclude that for over half the population auditory conceptualization matures naturally and is fully developed by fourth or fifth grade but that for a substantial segment of the population this skill does not develop spontaneously and remains deficient into adulthood. Regardless of the age of the individual, however, the Lindamoods contend that auditory-conceptualization function can be taught through direct, multisensory instruction.

CURRICULUM AND INSTRUCTION

The ADD program contains five developmental levels. The first level, called "Setting the Climate for Learning," is essentially an introduction to the concept of auditory perception; students are taught how to listen selectively and to make judgments about sounds. Activities include identifying environmental sounds, comparing sounds, and sequencing sounds.

The second curriculum level teaches students to identify and classify speech sounds. All sounds have been categorized and labeled on the basis of how the mouth is formed when the sounds are produced. Sixteen of the consonant sounds have been grouped in unvoiced/voiced pairs; /p/ and /b/, for example are paired and labeled "lip poppers"; /p/ is the "quiet brother" and /b/ is the "noisy brother." For vowels, which have more subtle characteristics in pronounciation, students are taught "to associate the physical sensation of making each sound, the appearance of the mouth when the sound is made, and the sound they hear" (Lindamood and Lindamood 1975, Book 1). Students are asked to think of the vowels as falling on a half circle moving from the front to the back of the mouth, depending upon placement of the tongue when a vowel is pronounced. The short /i/ sound, for instance, is produced with the tongue placed high in the front of the mouth.

At the next level, students learn to track sounds in nonsense words. Colored blocks are used to distinguish the various sound categories (color by itself has no meaning). The instructor might say, "Show me /zab/," and the student would place in sequence three blocks of different colors. If then asked, "Show me /zat/," the student would remove the last block and replace it with a different block of another color. In this way, simple syllables (CV, VC, and CVC) and complex syllables (CCV, VVC, CCVC, CVCC, and CCVCC) are taught.

Not until students have become proficient at encoding nonsense words in this manner, are letter symbols introduced. At this fourth level of the curriculum, students first use letters printed on tiles for spelling ac-

	Given Sound Pattern	Student's Label and Block Pattern*		Given Sound Pattern	Student's Label and Block Pattern
			"Show me	/ab/." (two different sounds)	"A smile /a/ and a lip popper"
					☐ ■
					(two blocks of different colors)
"Show me	/b/ /b/ /b/." (one sound repeated three times)	"three lip poppers" ☐ ☐ ☐ (three blocks of the same color)			
			"If that says /ab/, show me	/zab/." (same two sounds as in original pattern, with the *addition* of a new and different initial sound)	"A skinny sound came at the beginning." ▨ ☐ ■ (same two blocks as in original pattern, with the addition of a block of a third color at the beginning)
"Show me	/t/ /m/." (two different sounds)	"a tip tapper and a nose sound" ☐ ■ (two blocks of different colors)			
			"If that says show me	/zab/, /zaf/." (same initial and middle sounds as in previous pattern, with the *substitution* of a different final sound)	"The lip popper is gone and a lip cooler took its place." ▨ ☐ ▩ (same two initial and middle blocks as in previous pattern, with a block of a different color substituted for the final block)
"Show me	/s/ /s/ /g/." (one sound repeated two times, followed by one different sound)	"two skinny sounds and a scraper" ■ ■ ☐ (two blocks of the same color, followed by one block of a different color)			

*The block drawings are not intended to represent specific colors. They simply indicate the pattern of sameness or difference within each sequence.

Color-Encoding Isolated Sounds. The A.D.D. Program: Auditory Discrimination in Depth *by Charles H. Lindamood and Patricia C. Lindamood. (Reproduced with permission from DLM Teaching Resources, Allen, TX. Copyright 1975.)*

Color-Encoding Sounds in Syllables. The A.D.D. Program: Auditory Discrimination in Depth *by Charles H. Lindamood and Patricia C. Lindamood. (Reproduced with permission from DLM Teaching Resources, Allen, TX. Copyright 1975.)*

tivities and then progress to writing letters themselves. Real words are introduced at this level along with commercially available spelling programs. Students learn to sort out phonetically regular, or dependable, words from nonphonetic words. This allows them to concentrate on the irregular features of the latter type, according to the Lindamoods, and reduces the number of words that must be memorized.

Reading, or decoding, the fifth level of the ADD curriculum, may overlap with the fourth level and follows much the same sequence as spelling instruction, beginning with letter tiles and moving to written words. The curriculum systematically brings into play a three-way sensory feedback system from the ear, eye, and mouth to be used in monitoring and verifying sound–symbol correspondences. Verbal mediation is encouraged as a processing strategy at all levels of the program, with the expectation that through repeated practice the self-correction process will become internalized.

Minimal coverage is given to reading comprehension in the ADD teacher manuals, although recent correspondence from the Lindamood's clinic in California indicates that procedures that stimulate visual imagery have recently been developed by Nanci Bell (see Chapter 4, Reading Comprehension Instruction, p. 88). In the ADD manual the Lindamoods advocate using either linguistic or i.t.a. (Initial Teaching Alphabet) readers in the beginning reading stages and emphasize the importance of oral reading. For severely disabled readers, they suggest that the teacher first read the text aloud in order to model intonation, as well as to provide awareness of general content and vocabulary.

The ADD techniques are designed for classroom use with small, homogenous groups of students, although they can be applied in tutorial settings as well. The teacher uses a Socratic approach to instruction and through questioning leads students to discover the alphabetic principle for themselves (Howard 1982).

TEACHER TRAINING

Teacher training for the Lindamood ADD program is conducted in two five-day, nine-hour seminars. The first seminar teaches theory and demonstates treatment concepts and techniques. The second seminar, which usually follows immediately after the first, involves practical application of concepts and techniques. These seminars are offered at the Lindamood Language and Literacy Center in San Luis Obispo, California.

Alternatively, inservice training can be arranged; teachers who intend to conduct the inservice must participate in a two-week training workshop at the center. As the duration of training is much shorter, inservice training costs are considerably less than those of the Slingerland and Alphabetic phonics programs.

EVALUATION AND IMPLEMENTATION

Analyses of data on the effectiveness of the ADD program have yielded generally positive results. Marilyn Howard (1982), conducting joint pilot studies in Arco, Indiana and Santa Maria, California, found that average reading scores for children who had received ADD instruction as first graders rose by more than 30 percentile points over a five-year period. Robert Calfee (1976) demonstrated remarkable superiority for the ADD program over both the Sullivan and Gillingham-Stillman programs, as well as over a basal reader program, with 174 second-grade students in one school district.

A three-year study (INTRAC 1983) investigated the effects of incorporating the Lindamood program with the Ginn basal reader program in first- through third-grade classrooms by comparing academic progress in these classrooms to progress in classrooms using only the Ginn program. At the end of the first year, superior gains were evidenced in the experimental classrooms as compared to the control classrooms, not only in auditory conceptualization but also on the spelling, reading, and word attack subtests of the California Achievement Test (CAT). At the end of the second year of ADD training, students in the experimental classrooms increased their lead over the control subjects.

As a result of the favorable outcome for ADD instruction in the INTRAC study, the school board voted in the third year to provide inservice training for teachers and to include the ADD curriculum in all kindergarten through second-grade classrooms in the school district. Letters promoting the ADD program have been written by school principals, as well as college deans, testifying to the successful results of the progam with their students.

More recently, further positive evidence of the effectiveness of ADD has been provided in a study that analyzed program evaluation data collected over eleven years (Howard 1986). The study produced three major findings:

1. Students receiving ADD training in first grade made greater gains in word attack and reading achievement over the year and had higher reading scores in following years than students not receiving the training.
2. Kindergarten children trained in ADD techniques had higher word attack skills upon entering first grade than students not taught these techniques.
3. ADD training was equally effective with boys and girls.

CHAPTER

14

The Slingerland Program

BACKGROUND AND RATIONALE

The Slingerland Program was developed in 1960 by Beth Slingerland as an adaption of the Orton-Gillingham approach to be used with whole classes of students. It began in the Pacific Northwest and has its headquarters in Bellevue, Washington. Hundreds of Slingerland classrooms now exist on the West Coast and more are springing up in other areas of the United States.

The program was designed as preventive instruction for children who have been identified by the Slingerland Screening Tests as having "specific language disability" and therefore at risk for reading failure. The tests are usually administered at the end of kindergarten or beginning of first grade. Children so identified receive Slingerland instruction in place of the traditional language arts curriculum; most remain in Slingerland classrooms for at least two years.

Like the Orton-Gillingham, the Slingerland approach is based on the premise that language depends upon intersensory functioning. Multisensory activities are incorporated into all levels of the program to promote the development of automatic visual, auditory, and kinesthetic associations.

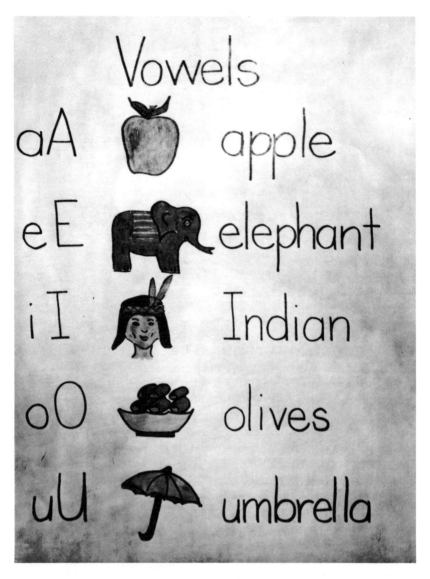

Slingerland Wall Card. Photograph from A Multi-Sensory Approach to Language Arts for Specific Language Disability Children *by Beth H. Slingerland. (Reproduced with permission from Educators Publishing Service, Cambridge, MA. Copyright 1971.)*

CURRICULUM AND INSTRUCTION

Slingerland training begins with learning to write, as described in the section on spelling instruction in Chapter 8, Spelling Instruction (pp. 96 to 97). Children learn to form letters in manuscript, first by tracing, copying, writing in the air, and writing from memory, while saying the letter names. The order of letter introduction is arbitrary, although the teacher's manual provides a list of ten consonants to be taught, along with a vowel, in the first several months. Each letter is shown on a wall card in upper and lower case, with a picture of a key word, as well as the written word itself, for example, house for *h*. An alphabet flashcard is also provided for each letter and used in daily practice of sound-symbol associations.

After learning to write a letter, the students are taught the letter sound along with its key word. For reinforcement, the teacher calls upon individual children to name the letter, name the key word, and give the letter sound. Both unison and individual response is used in the Slingerland program. In answering individually, the child usually stands up in order that the rest of the class can observe, as well as hear, his or her response.

The Slingerland curriculum is divided into two components: the Auditory Approach and the Visual Approach. In the Auditory Approach, which leads to blending and then spelling, the stimulus is presented orally. The teacher says each letter sound and asks individual children to name the letter while forming it in the air, then to name its key word and give its sound. In this way, auditory and kinesthetic modalities apparently are linked. The teacher then holds up an alphabet card and has the class repeat the procedure in unison, linking the visual and auditory modalities.

Blending is introduced with oral activities, using a pocket chart for kinesthetic reinforcement. The teacher pronounces a c-v-c word, for example, *hat;* the class repeats the word; an individual child produces the initial sound /h/, gives its letter name, and places the corresponding letter in the pocket chart. The child repeats the word, pronounces the vowel sound before naming the vowel and places the letter next to the first, and so on. Once pupils are able to do this, as well as to form the letters correctly on lined paper, writing accompanies the pocket chart activity.

In the Visual Approach, which leads to reading, the stimulus is presented in its written form. Decoding, referred to as "unlocking words," however, is not taught until blending and spelling skills taught in the Auditory Approach are "reasonably automatic and functional" (Slingerland 1971), usually in the second semester of first grade. Decoding instruction begins with c-v-c words. Students are asked to pronounce the initial consonant, then the vowel, then to blend the two, then to pronounce the final consonant, and finally to say the whole word. Once they are able to decode letter by letter, the students are taught to look first for the vowel in each word and to follow the procedures for identifying that vowel sound. For example, in decoding the word "map," the student would say, "*a,* apple, /a/, map." Slingerland (1971) maintains that consonant blends "usu-

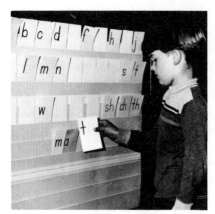 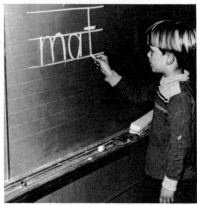

Spelling Activities in the Slingerland Program. Photographs from A Multi-Sensory Approach to language Arts for Specific Language Disability Children *by Beth H. Slingerland. (Reproduced with permission from Educators Publishing Service. Copyright 1971.)*

ally fall into place" and need not be taught in isolation. However, vowel digraphs and vowel-consonant digraphs are taught as units, as are inflectional endings, such as -*ed* and -*ing*.

Text reading is taught initially via a whole word approach, usually with whichever basal reader program is used in the school. It can begin, according to Slingerland, at the same time as it is introduced in the other first-grade classrooms and is conducted in small groups. A considerable amount of lesson time is spent on "preparation for reading" in which students practice recognizing and reading words and phrases from the text. The teacher writes a list of new words on the chalkboard and the students learn, in performing various activities, to recognize the word, pronounce the word, and identify its meaning. Towards this last end, the teacher might, for example, ask a student to find the word in the list that "tells the name of a girl" (Jill) or "tells what children do" (swim). Phrases are taught in the same way, and fluency and intonation are emphasized, with the teacher modeling by reading aloud.

The teacher structures the text reading by calling attention to the phrases, for example: "The next three words go together. Read them to yourselves." As previously mentioned in Chapter 7, the teacher guides comprehension by asking questions such as "What three words tell where the pony ran?" ("to the barn").

Although the basic Slingerland curriculum is designed for the first two primary grades and is described in two corresponding teacher guides (Books 1 and 2), a third year curriculum has been developed for Slingerland students who need further support after second grade, as well as older reading disabled students who were not picked up earlier (Book 3). Cursive writing is introduced in this curriculum.

TEACHER TRAINING

Training as a Slingerland teacher involves participation in a four week teacher training course. This training usually takes place during the summer within summer school classrooms established for children identified in the Slingerland program as having a language learning disability and provides graduate credits at an affiliated college or university. Staff members from the Slingerland Institute or Slingerland teachers within the school district serve as teacher trainers. The program is coordinated by a certified Slingerland director, who has had two years of Slingerland instruction, plus a third year of classroom supervision, followed by experience as a Slingerland staff teacher.

Dolores Ballesteros and Nancy Royal (1981) describe the organization of a Slingerland summer school training program in a large school district. The program director is responsible for the overall management of the training program, which includes evaluating the training staff. He or she also gives lectures to the teacher-participants on language development, reading and language disabilities, phonics, and multisensory techniques. Staff teachers must be well versed in the Slingerland techniques and must be approved by the Slingerland Institute. Each staff teacher works with fifteen teacher-participants, demonstrating teaching techniques within a classroom and meeting with teachers for discussion and daily lesson planning. Besides attending lectures and classroom demonstrations, each teacher-participant works daily with an individual child, under the supervision of a staff teacher. A clerical staff member is hired when the number of teacher-participants exceeds forty-five.

School district expenses for a Slingerland summer school training program include staff salaries, minimal supply costs for children's materials and minimal printing costs, in addition to a teacher-participant service charge to the Slingerland Institute for in-service staff and Slingerland materials. Teacher-participants usually pay for teacher's materials and tuition for university credit where it is available (Ballesteros and Royal 1981). All Slingerland training programs must be planned through the Slingerland Institute in Bellevue, Washington. Summer schools are held only in districts providing administrative support for teachers interested in Slingerland instruction.

PROGRAM EVALUATION AND IMPLEMENTATION

The Slingerland method has been enthusiastically received in a large number of school districts throughout the country, particularly in the Pacific Northwest, where it originated, and in California. In many cases, parents have been instrumental in starting Singerland programs and in some instances have even threatened to file suit unless their children were provided with this instruction (Lovitt and DeMier 1984). Ballesteros and Royal (1981) described how the program served as a voluntary magnet for school racial integration in Southern California: Slingerland classes were established in high-minority schools in the San Diego area with two-thirds enrollment space reserved for nonminority students from the district in which parents had requested this instruction. Moreover, through parental petition Slingerland classes were established in this area all the way through twelfth grade level!

Considerable research has addressed the question of program effectiveness. John Litcher and Leonard Roberge (1979) conducted a three-year study with first grade children receiving Slingerland instruction, comparing their year end achievement with matched control children in other schools. They reported significantly higher achievement for the Slingerland students. However, because they did not describe the instruction provided to the control subjects the comparison is less meaningful.

Beverly Wolf (1985) conducted an ex post facto analysis of first- to second-grade gain scores on the Metropolitan Achievement Test (MAT) of children in Slingerland classes, some of whom were considered to be language disabled, as determined by the Slingerland Screening Tests, and some of whom were not. These scores were compared to those of children in conventional classrooms who met the same criteria. Instruction in the conventional classrooms, which served as the control treatment, was not described in detail, but appears to have been an eclectic basal reader approach. Thus two experimental groups received Slingerland instruction, those with "specific language disability" (SLD) and those without SLD, and two control groups received conventional instruction, one SLD, the other non-SLD. The outcome of the analysis indicated that Slingerland instruction produced significantly greater gains than conventional instruction on the language section of the MAT (listening comprehension; punctuation and capitalization; usage, grammar, and syntax; spelling; and study skills) for both SLD and non-SLD students. On the reading section (word and sentence reading; vocabulary; literal, inferential, and evaluative comprehension) the advantage of Slingerland training over conventional instruction approached but did not achieve significance; however, scores of the Slingerland students were less variable than those of the conventional group. The superiority of Slingerland instruction over conventional instruction was not evidenced in the reading scores, on the other hand, for the non-SLD children.

Another ex post facto investigation (McCulloch 1985) compared California Achievement Test (CAT) scores of 15 SLD children who received three years of Slingerland training with 15 SLD children who had been taught in conventional classrooms during the first three grades. Statistical analyses demonstrated significantly higher reading and language scores for the Slingerland trained children. Spelling scores, in contrast, did not reveal significant between-group differences. The study's author, Clara McCulloch, suggests that this latter finding reflects the nature of the CAT spelling task which requires picking out misspelled words in sentences, virtually a proof-reading task. She explains that because Slingerland students are taught to spell using an auditory approach and to read using a visual approach, the CAT spelling task runs counter to their training experience and may not tap their true spelling ability.

School-wide and district-wide evaluation studies of the Slingerland program have yielded generally positive results. For example, a study conducted in 1980 by the Bureau of Child Educational Services (BOCES) in South Huntington, New York, determined that by third grade Slingerland students had achieved reading gains equal to children in regular classrooms, although they did not reach the same reading level. The Slingerland Institute has stated emphatically that the achievement levels of SLD students should not be compared to those of normal students, but instead with expected year to year gains, as in this study.

One of the disconcerting observations I have made in reviewing the school evaluation studies, as well as in school visits, is that Slingerland instruction has not always been sufficient; in some schools children diagnosed as learning disabled are placed in a resource room. It would be important to know the differentiating characteristics of these children in order to determine whether they need more intensive or more individualized instruction than the Slingerland program offers or a different type of instruction altogether.

CHAPTER 15

Recipe for Reading

BACKGROUND AND RATIONALE

Recipe for Reading is another adaption of the Orton-Gillingham approach (Gillingham and Stillman 1960) and, like the Orton-Gillingham, is designed for one-to-one tutorial use. It was developed in the 1950s by Nina Traub and first used in Ossining, New York, with parents serving as tutors for learning disabled children in the community. Because of its success, funding was obtained in the early 1970s to place the program in five Ossining elementary schools (Traub 1982).

The Traub method applies a synthetic phonics approach, teaching individual letter sounds in isolation before introducing syllables or words. All teaching follows a part-to-whole progression.

In the instructor's manual (Traub and Bloom 1975), Mrs. Traub states that students who appear to have learning disabilities should be individually diagnosed and receive carefully planned individualized instruction. She maintains that learning disabilities vary among children, reflecting problems in visual, auditory, or tactile domains, and that instruction should be geared to modality strengths.

Although the term multisensory does not appear in the manual, the use of visual, auditory, and kinesthetic reinforcement techniques is encouraged throughout the program. Traub developed a sequence for introducing letter sounds based on their visual, auditory, and kinesthetic characteristics.

CURRICULUM AND INSTRUCTION

The Traub method is designed for first- through third-grade students to be delivered on a one-to-one basis outside the classroom in half-hour sessions five days a week. In developing Recipe for Reading, Traub has greatly simplified the Orton-Gillingham curriculum. Her teacher's manual (Traub and Bloom 1975) is clearly written, easy to follow, and relatively short. A curriculum sequence chart is printed on the inside cover.

Instruction begins by introducing seven consonants (hard *c* and *g*, *d, m, l, h,* and *t*) and two vowels (*a* and *o*). Explaining the rationale for her selection of these letters, Traub states in the manual that some letters are learned and written more easily than others. As examples, she maintains that *c, o, a,* and *d* have the same basic kinesthetic formations (circle to the left), hard *c* and *g* "seem to be among the easiest sounds perceived by the ear," *d* and *m* are two of the first sounds made by infants ("da-da," "ma-ma"). *D* and *b* "are introduced at a considerable distance from each other, because they are the pair that are most commonly reversed and confused."

Each letter to be learned is first presented on a large piece of oak tag, written in one-inch thick strokes. The teacher gives the letter sound and then writes the letter. The child traces the letter and then writes it independently. When the child has done this successfully, the teacher says the letter name.

Both manuscript and cursive letter formations are taught in the Traub method. Special lined paper is provided to designate orientation points in letter formation. Each writing line is divided into four parallel lines. Letters with no stems should fill the space between the two middle lines, called "the little red house." Upward letter stems should touch the top line ("the attic") and downward stems the bottom line ("the basement"). Directional cues for letter formations are provided at the top of each page—a bat and a ball for letters such as *b,* that turn to the right, and a drum and drumstick for those turning to the left. Many multisensory techniques are suggested for the student who has difficulty with letter formations, for example, walking on a letter formed with masking tape on the floor, forming a letter with rolls of clay and then tracing it with eyes open and eyes shut, and writing in the air ("sky writing").

Spelling precedes reading in the Traub approach. After the student has learned the sound and name for each of the first nine letters and is able to write each of these letters, the student is taught to spell c-v-c words with these letters. The teacher dictates words without the student's having seen the words in print. The student repeats the word, spells it aloud, and then writes it while spelling it aloud (simultaneous oral spelling). If the student has difficulty, he or she is asked to listen for the first sound and give its letter name as the teacher says the word, separating each phoneme. This procedure is repeated with the middle vowel and final consonant.

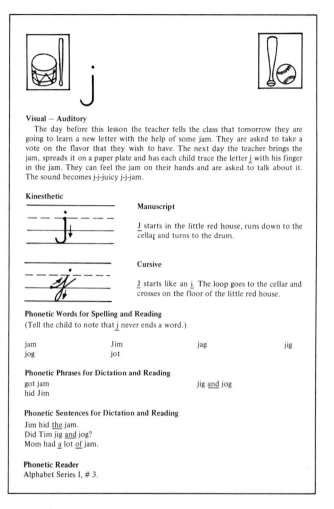

Visual — Auditory

The day before this lesson the teacher tells the class that tomorrow they are going to learn a new letter with the help of some jam. They are asked to take a vote on the flavor that they wish to have. The next day the teacher brings the jam, spreads it on a paper plate and has each child trace the letter j with his finger in the jam. They can feel the jam on their hands and are asked to talk about it. The sound becomes j-j-juicy j-j-jam.

Kinesthetic

Manuscript

J starts in the little red house, runs down to the cellar and turns to the drum.

Cursive

J starts like an i. The loop goes to the cellar and crosses on the floor of the little red house.

Phonetic Words for Spelling and Reading

(Tell the child to note that j never ends a word.)

jam	Jim	jag	jig
jog	jot		

Phonetic Phrases for Dictation and Reading

got jam   jig and jog
hid Jim

Phonetic Sentences for Dictation and Reading

Jim hid the jam.
Did Tim jig and jog?
Mom had a lot of jam.

Phonetic Reader
Alphabet Series I, # 3.

Lesson from Recipe for Reading *by Nina Traub with Frances Bloom. (Reproduced with permission from Educators Publishing Service, Cambridge, MA. Copyright 1975.)*

The manual tells the teacher to dictate more naturally "as the child's auditory discrimination improves" (Traub and Bloom 1975).

After the student spells words, he is asked to read them as printed on flash cards ("phonetic word cards"), rather than in his own writing. If the student has trouble reading a word, the teacher places cards representing each letter ("phonetic sound cards") under the word and has the student say each letter sound. Traub suggests many blending techniques but, like Gillingham and Stillman (1960), emphasizes first blending the initial consonant and following vowel, for example, *ba-t,* rather than the vowel and final consonant, as in the phonic-linguistic approach (e.g., *b-at*), which she claims encourages wrong directionality.

Once the student can spell several words, the teacher dictates phrases or short sentences for the student to write, providing the spelling for any nonphonetic word. Maintaining that auditory memory deficiency may present a problem in sentence dictation, Traub recommends tasks for memory training.

After writing sentences, the student reads these sentences from "phonetic sentence cards" and when ready, graduates to reading "phonetic storybooks," following the same procedures. In addition to these storybooks, Traub provides a list of phonetic readers from other publishers for supplementary reading. She suggests that teachers alternate oral reading with students to model fluency and expression and that they discuss the passage content with students.

Recognizing the low interest level of most phonetic readers, Traub recommends reading other materials aloud to the student to develop comprehension skills. She suggests asking the student to listen for the answer to a particular question as the text is read.

Having the student dictate his or her own stories is another suggested activity in Recipe for Reading. The teacher types the story, which is then made into a book for the child and others to read, much like the language experience approach. Traub maintains that this activity improves verbal expression and helps build a sight vocabulary. She also recommends using Dolch flash cards[1] for building sight vocabulary development.

Briefly, the Traub curriculum moves from one-syllable words, to two-syllable compound words (e.g., pigpen) to two-syllable phonetic words (dislike). In the last instance, the student first reads the individual syllables on cards and then puts them together to make words. All letter sounds or groups of letter sounds are introduced one by one: initial consonant blends, three letter word endings (e.g., *ing, ank*), long vowel sound with "magic *e*", vowel digraphs, vowel-consonant combinations, diphthongs, nonphonetic word parts, such as *igh,* and common suffixes, such as *ing, tion,* and *sion.* Only a few basic spelling rules are emphasized, such as when to double final consonants. A special section on affixes and word roots is provided for older students.

Daily lessons begin with drill on previously learned letter sounds. Then new material is presented and taught as previously described. Depending on the student's ability level, word reading, sentence reading, and story book reading follow in order. Lastly, phonetic word games are played to reinforce learning.

---

[1]The Dolch Basic Sight Vocabulary Cards (Dolch 1952) which contain 220 of the most frequently encountered English words.

Each student's work is dated and retained in a folder, and his progress carefully recorded. A count is kept of all words learned. Traub emphasizes the importance of making students aware of their progress. For younger children, particularly, she recommends ending lessons with an activity at which they are sure to succeed and acknowledging their success with some sign of approval. By way of additional encouragement, a list of all the books a student has read is included in his folder.

An addendum to the Recipe for Reading manual is currently being written, which will include lesson plans, games, and mastery tests. Student workbooks to accompany the program will also soon be available.

TEACHER TRAINING

All training for Recipe for Reading teachers or tutors was conducted by Mrs. Traub, the program's author, until her death. Since then, her colleague, Mrs. Connie Russo, has carried on the program and conducted the teacher training. The following description of the teacher training program was provided by Mrs. Russo via telephone.

Training is usually done within a public school in daily, five-hour sessions over a two week period. It is best arranged during the summer when children are attending classes for remedial instruction. The first two hours are devoted to lecture. In the next two hours each teacher trainee applies the knowledge acquired from the lecture by tutoring two public school students for one hour each under supervision. The last hour involves a sharing and pulling together of all that has been learned that day among the fifteen or so teacher trainees.

When training is conducted during the school year, it is usually condensed into six hours of lecture without the tutoring practicum because of problems with classroom pull-out time. However, supervised tutoring experience is arranged individually for each teacher trainee during the year.

EVALUATION AND IMPLEMENTATION

A federally funded validation study, reported by Mrs. Traub (1982), was carried out in 1976 by the MAGI Educational Service on the initial school implementation of Recipe for Reading in five Ossining elementary schools. Results of this study showed that second grade Ossining students tutored with Recipe for Reading made significantly greater improvement in reading and spelling, as measured by posttests, than a control group of second grade students from another district tutored using a different remedial method that was not described. Unfortunately, since the tests administered yield only total reading grade equivalents, it is not possible to ascertain which subskills (decoding, vocabulary, or comprehension) are most influenced by the Traub method.

As a result of this validation study, Ossining received a federal IV-C grant to continue and expand the use of Recipe for Reading. Mrs. Traub (1982) states that subsequent to the program's implementation in Ossining, twenty-six different school districts had received similar grants to replicate the Ossining program and that she had trained the staff in these schools. She reports positive effects of Recipe for Reading, as measured by year to year comparison studies on student achievement conducted in several of these districts. One district cited the program's cost effectiveness, maintaining that personnel was the highest expense and that expense for materials was low. Another district cited enhanced motivation and improved attitude toward reading among students receiving Recipe for Reading instruction.

The Traub method is most often used within the special education framework, both in self-contained classrooms and in resource rooms. However, it is sometimes used in regular classrooms with children appearing to be at high risk for reading failure. Though designed for one-to-one instruction, Mrs. Russo maintains that the method is ideal for small groups of as many as five students. The Rippowam-Cisqua School, a private school in Bedford, New York, uses Recipe for Reading as a beginning reading program with all students. An expansion of the curriculum is being written currently for upper elementary, junior high and high school students.

CHAPTER

16

Project Read (Enfield and Greene)

BACKGROUND AND RATIONALE

Project Read was developed in 1969 by Mary Lee Enfield and Victoria Greene for the public school district in Bloomington, Minnesota, in response to the growing number of children who were not benefitting from the basal reading program used in the district. It began as a three year experimental program to deliver direct, systematic phonics instruction within regular classrooms to students performing below the 25th percentile in reading and spelling. The major goals of the program were to provide cost effective reading instruction to students who were not learning in the district's reading program, to increase coordination between regular classroom instruction and remedial instruction, and to avoid the stigma of removal from the mainstream (Enfield 1976). The authors consider the program an alternative as well as a remedial approach to reading instruction (Enfield and Greene 1981).

Project Read is now being used with students in grades one through six who are functioning at the lowest reading levels, as well as with students identified as learning disabled. Though designed for the classroom teacher, the program may be used effectively in a resource center (Arkes 1986). Extensions of the program, covering reading comprehension and written expression, as well as phonology, are appropriate for intermediate and secondary students who are weak in these areas.

CURRICULUM AND INSTRUCTION

Project Read curriculum comprises three phases. Phase I instruction focuses on phonics, Phase II on reading comprehension, and Phase III on written expression. Phase I is essentially a modification of the Gillingham-Stillman model of systematic, multisensory phonics instruction. Originally designed for grades one through three, Phase I has since been extended through grade nine. Instruction in basic phonics knowledge for grades one through three is outlined in a teacher's guide (Greene and Enfield 1985a). The guide provides a systematic sequence of skills and concepts that are covered in a series of sixty lessons, each of which may span several days or even a week of instruction. Specific techniques, many of which are multisensory, are described for teaching these skills and concepts. These include tracing letters in a sand tray (called the memory box), in the air, on a shag rug, a table, or a chalkboard. Raised letters are provided for showing directionality of confusable letters. Mouth positions are stressed in teaching consonant sounds, for example, for *b*, a voiced explosion of air, for *t*, a tongue bounce, for *m*, mouth closed. Finger puppets and key words are mnemonics suggested for teaching vowels, and children are given practice in identifying the vowels from among the other letters in the alphabet sequence. Long and short vowel markings are taught in the first lesson.

Each lesson introduces a new phonic element, such as a letter sound, and a particular concept, for instance, the fact that vowels have a significant value for building words. A lesson begins with review of previously learned material that includes both decoding and encoding practice. Hand signals are used to direct unison response. The teacher flashes letter cards and the students say the letter sounds; the teacher says the sounds and the students write the letter symbols. Next, new sounds are introduced and reinforced with multisensory techniques. Students then build words or syllables with letter cards and decode them. Various techniques for sound blending are described in the teacher's guide. Spelling practice follows with students saying the letter sound as they write each letter.

Oral reading is the last activity of each lesson. The program has incorporated the *SRA Basic Reading* linguistic series (Rasmussen and Goldberg 1976) for this purpose, although alternative materials are suggested in some of the lessons. Students are taught to follow along with a finger or pencil while reading and, if they have difficulty decoding, to trace over the particular letter or letters "to unlock the sound" (Greene and Enfield 1985a). Oral reading involves both "reinforcement reading," where the material is usually phonetically regular and students are expected to have little decoding difficulty, and "stretch reading," where the material may include unfamiliar words. Irregular words contained in reinforcement reading material are taught separately. In stretch reading the teacher supplies any words that may be beyond the students skill level.

Three categories of words are distinguished in Project Read: "green words" which are phonetically regular for both decoding and encoding (e.g., cat); "yellow words" which are regular for decoding but follow spelling generalizations for encoding (e.g., back); and "red words" which are irregular for both decoding and encoding (e.g., the).

A continuation of Phase I for students in fourth through ninth grades focuses on vocabulary development by teaching affixes and common word roots. The curriculum is outlined in a second Phase I teacher guide, referred to as the Affix Guide (Greene and Enfield 1981). The guide presents a unique approach to unlocking word meaning; rather than drawing attention to word roots, which may be elements too obscure to bear apparent meaning (for example, *dict* in "unpredictable") students are taught to look for known parts (in this case *predict*), which are referred to as "word foundations." After identifying the known foundation, the attending affixes are isolated and identified.

Another creative aspect of Greene and Enfield's curriculum is their application of the concept of compression to the understanding of affixed words. Students learn that these words actually represent phrases, for example, *unpredictable* equals "cannot be predicted." The teacher's guide presents pairs of sentences, one containing such a phrase, the other the corresponding affixed word. It also provides sentences that can be used for demonstration and reinforcement in dictation exercises, using the affixed words in meaningful context. A spelling guide incorporating a structured phonics approach is also included in the Project Read materials (Enfield and Greene 1985). The guide provides the teacher with valuable information about English spelling patterns and rules. It takes into consideration three relevant aspects of English graphemes: their origin (e.g., Anglo Saxon, Latin), their frequency, and their placement in words. In terms of frequency, Enfield and Greene maintain that teaching the least frequently encountered spellings for a particular phoneme first—for example, *ue* before *ew*—helps students learn to sort and classify words according to spelling patterns.

The syllable is the unit of emphasis in this spelling guide. According to Greene and Enfield, all syllables in the English language fall into one of seven categories: closed, open, vowel team, vowel-consonant-final *e*, diphthong, final consonant *le*, and vowel controlled by *r*. They stress the fact that the type of syllable determines the sound of the vowel or vowels it contains.

Phase II of Project Read focuses on reading comprehension and vocabulary development and begins when a student has mastered basic decoding skills, usually toward the end of first grade. However, major emphasis on comprehension instruction takes place in grades four through six. The curriculum is outlined in a teacher's guide (Greene and Enfield 1985b) which has incorporated instructional materials from other publish-

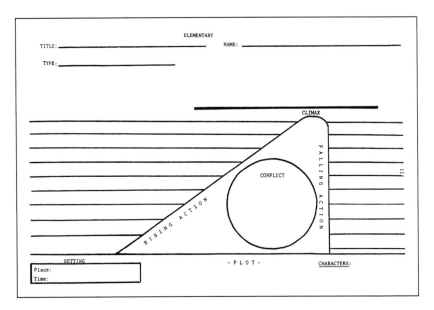

Diagram of Story Form from There's a Skeleton in Every Closet, Teacher Text *by Victoria E. Greene and Mary Lee Enfield. (Reproduced with permission from the authors. Copyright 1976.)*

ers for teaching reading comprehension skills, for example, the McGraw Hill Reading for Concepts series and the Barnell Loft Specific Skills Series. Most of these materials are nonfiction.

The guide distinguishes two levels of text analysis and presents a sequence of comprehension skills within each level. At the literal level these skills include identifying the subject of the text, selecting and defining unfamiliar words, noting punctuation and understanding its purpose, and determining whether the text material is fiction, nonfiction, or procedural (telling how to do something). At the interpretive level, the skills include identifying and sequencing the information in the text (either key facts or key procedural steps), finding the supporting details, making inferences, and drawing conclusions. Students also are taught to outline the organizational form of a text.

Multisensory activities are suggested to reinforce the concepts being taught. For example, having students write key facts on paper cut-out keys and paste the keys in the margins, pointing to the facts as written in the text, or having students feel an object hidden in a paper bag and make assumptions about that object from touch.

The major focus in the inference unit of the curriculum is on teaching students to look for clues in the text that lead to or support assumptions about the content. Toward this end the teacher may make an inferential statement and ask students to find the clues in the text that lead to this inference or the teacher may ask an inferential question for students to answer and indicate the clues that led to their answer.

An additional teacher text (Greene and Enfield 1983) has been written for teaching older children with language learning problems. This guide deals with genre and style of literature, as well as emphasizing the structure of text. Considerable attention is devoted to understanding story form. Model diagrams are provided for demonstrating the structure of a story plot (conflict, rising action, climax, falling action), and students are taught to fill in the appropriate information on a diagram after analyzing a story selection.

Phase III of Project Read encompasses instruction in written expression, provided systematically and incorporating multisensory techniques. Handwriting instruction, however, is not included in the program. The focus in this phase is on teaching sentence structure and paragraph development. Instruction moves from basic sentence structure (simple sentences) to complex sentences. Students are taught to diagram sentences; they spend considerable time at this activity. Concepts are practiced in creative writing experiences. Phase III extends from the end of grade one through grade nine and may be used as an alternative to the regular English program in grades five through nine (Arkes 1986).

TEACHER TRAINING

In the early stages of Project Read, training was carried out by ten former classroom teachers who had learned the program. Using demonstration and observational methods, they in turn taught the program in schools to elementary teachers as they worked with groups of poorly achieving students in their classrooms. At the end of two or three weeks, the classroom teacher took over full responsibility for the program, supported by periodic visits from the project staff for further observation, feedback, and demonstration as needed.

At the present time, half-day workshops of five days each are held during the summer in Bloomington at the Project Read Teacher Training Institute. Each workshop is devoted to one of three instructional areas: phonology, reading comprehension, or written expression. Training for workshop attendees continues in the following school year with demonstration and observation of the program in their respective classrooms in the district.

EVALUATION AND IMPLEMENTATION

The first evaluation of Project Read was conducted by Mary Lee Enfield in 1976 as a pilot study. An experimental group of forty-five children in grades one through three, fifteen at each grade level, who were reading below the 25th percentile, received Project Read instruction. As compared to a matched control group of children from another school district who did not receive Project Read instruction, the experimental subjects made significantly greater gains on measures of reading and spelling achievement. Because of these favorable results, the Bloomington school board mandated the implementation of Project Read in all first- through third-grade classrooms in the district.

A second evaluation was conducted on the initial three years of the program as implemented district-wide (Enfield 1976). Data were analyzed from a battery of reading and spelling tests administered to a random sample of 665 students in grades one through three who had participated in Project Read. Results of the analyses indicated the following:

1. significant gains for Project Read students on most of the tests given;
2. a significant reduction in the number of children requiring tutoring services at the end of the three year period;
3. greater yearly gains in reading for Project Read students than for children in previous tutoring programs;
4. a significant reduction in teacher cost per pupil for Project Read students as compared to students in tutoring programs;
5. a district-wide reduction of students falling below grade level in reading after two years of Project Read implementation.

One of the major limitations of the study, as Enfield herself has pointed out, was the lack of a control group. She also acknowledges the possibility of a Hawthorne effect (performance enhancement) due to the novelty of the program. More recently, Enfield and Greene evaluated the progress of students in grades two, four, and six of the Bloomington public schools who were receiving Project Read instruction (Enfield and Greene 1983). Separate evaluations were conducted on results of district-wide standardized testing in reading and spelling for non-learning disabled students in the Project Read program and students classified as learning disabled who received Project Read instruction. Both evaluations indicated that Project Read students were performing above 75 percent of their achievement potential (estimated on the basis of IQ). Enfield and Greene maintain that this performance level represents significant improvement for these students who were otherwise functioning in the bottom quartile of their class. Their claim, however, must be regarded as being based on subjective judgment.

Project Read is being used increasingly in public school districts around the country: Portland, Oregon; Irvine, California; Tampa, Florida, to name just a few. According to Dr. Enfield (personal communication), an enthusiastic leader is needed to convince the school administration to undertake a pilot study. In some instances leadership has come from a motivated teacher.

An elementary school in Old Greenwich, Connecticut recently installed Project Read in its first two grades. Four classroom teachers and the reading specialist attended the summer phonology workshop in Bloomington and began using the program the following year with the lowest achieving students in their classrooms. Despite the lack of on-site supervision from the Project Read training staff, these teachers apparently gained enough confidence in their proficiency with the method to train other teachers in the school to use it.

CHAPTER
17

DISTAR

BACKGROUND AND RATIONALE

The Direct Instruction Model, which became known as DISTAR (Direct Instructional System of Teaching Arithmetic and Reading), was developed by Wesley Becker and Siegfried Engelmann at the University of Oregon. It was officially launched in 1968 as one of nine instructional models to be used in Project Follow-Through, a U.S. Government-sponsored project to evaluate the effectiveness of promising educational programs for disadvantaged children in the first three grades.

Four basic assumptions form the theoretical rationale for the DISTAR model (Becker 1977). First, all children, regardless of background and developmental readiness, can be taught, and teachers must be held accountable for student failure. Second, basic skills acquisition underlies all successful learning; for children who are socio-economically deprived, direct teaching of these skills is essential. Third, disadvantaged children generally lag behind advantaged students in basic skills acquisition due to the existing academic structure in most schools. The fourth assumption is that in order to close the achievement gap, disadvantaged youngsters must be taught more within the allotted instructional time than advantaged children.

Though originally designed for disadvantaged children, DISTAR has been used to teach children with a variety of constitutional handicaps, including learning disabilities. Writing in 1977, Norris Haring, Barbara Bateman, and Douglas Carnine stated:

> DISTAR's approach is representative of a growing trend in special educa-
> tion that shifts some attention from the child's strengths, weaknesses, or
> special etiology to an individualized remediation program for the *tasks* the
> child must learn.

Elsewhere in the same chapter, these strong advocates of Direct Instruction wrote:

> DISTAR's conceptualization encompasses all essential aspects of the teach-
> ing process—analyzing concepts, programming, teaching per se, class-
> room management, educational materials, and evaluation. It has de-
> veloped a way of analyzing tasks that isolates the general concept or skill to
> be taught, and a way to program in which this general case is presented so
> impecccably that every child can learn it. It has techniques for teaching the
> general case and strategies for classroom management.

CURRICULUM AND INSTRUCTION

Becker (1977) outlined seven essential instructional components of
the DISTAR model: (1) teaching general cases in order that learning can be
generalized from selected examples to broader instances; (2) higher
teacher-student ratio; (3) carefully structured daily curriculum; (4) rapid-
paced, teacher-directed, small-group instruction with a high number of
teacher/student interactions; (5) positive reinforcement; (6) carefully
trained and supervised teaching staff; and (7) biweekly performance monitoring by means of criterion-referenced tests.

A particularly discriminating feature of DISTAR is that all instruction follows a script. The presentation books (flip-books) provide exact
wording and precise directions for everything the teacher says and does in
each lesson. Instruction is conducted in small groups with students seated
in a semicircle close to the teacher in order to be able to see the one-inch
printed letters and words in the teacher presentation books. The proxim-
ity additionally helps the teacher to monitor student response, much of
which is done in unison. Teachers use hand signals, for example, a hand
drop, a clap, a point, or other cue, to indicate the type and timing of the
responses required. The presentation books ensure that all concepts
deemed relevant by the program's developers are taught and practiced by
the students. They include correction procedures and scripts for antici-
pated student errors.

DISTAR (Engelmann and Bruner 1983) is published by Science
Research Associates, Inc. and is now formally referred to as SRA's Direct
Instruction Programs. The programs provide instruction in reading, lan-
guage, spelling, and arithmetic and cover grade levels one through six.

The language program has three levels. The first level is for preschool and primary students and focuses on teaching the language of instruction used in school, building vocabulary, developing oral language skills, and establishing the foundation for logical thinking. The second level builds a language foundation for reading comprehension, emphasizing reasoning skills, and teaches following directions and the meanings of words and sentences. The third level focuses on sentence analysis, both spoken and written, and deals with mechanics, as well as informational content.

The reading program (Reading Mastery) has six levels; only levels I and II, which extend from preschool through second grade, will be discussed here. Both decoding and comprehension are taught from the very beginning.

In Reading Mastery I, letters are referred to as sounds; in Reading Mastery II, letter names are taught. Prereading activities start with teaching the pronunciations of letter sounds. Diagrams are presented to teach the distinction between continuous sounds (e.g., /s/, /m/, /r/, certain digraphs, and all vowels) and stop sounds (e.g., /b/, /d/, /t/). Games are played to promote sequencing skills and to teach understanding of cue words, such as "first" and "next." Oral blending activities begin in the first lesson and continue through the prereading lessons. Children are taught the difference between sounding out words (saying the letter sounds slowly) and pronouncing the words (saying them fast); the teacher uses hand signals in directing these activities. Rhyming activities are introduced to help children learn to blend initial sounds with word endings. Association between sounds and letter symbols is reinforced in take-home activities.

Letter sounds are introduced slowly in Reading Mastery I, about one every three to four lessons. Reading begins when six sounds have been learned. Each new sound to be taught is presented in a word; this word is used throughout the remainder of the program as a mnemonic device to cue the letter sound.

When new words are introduced, children are instructed first to sound out each word and then to say it fast. Irregular words, for example, *is, was,* are also initially taught in this way, with the teacher providing the correct pronounciation. It is felt that treating irregular words in this manner, rather than teaching them as "sight" words, emphasizes their stable spellings. All words learned become part of the students' reading vocabulary and are incorporated first in simple sentences and later in stories.

A modified orthography is used in the early stages of the DISTAR reading program and phased out by the middle of Reading Mastery II. The modification is meant to compensate for the unbalanced ratio of sounds to symbols in the English language and to increase the number of words that can be read as "regular" words, as well as to highlight differences between visually similar letters. The major features of this orthography include printing silent letters (e.g., *e* in made, *i* in maid) smaller, plac-

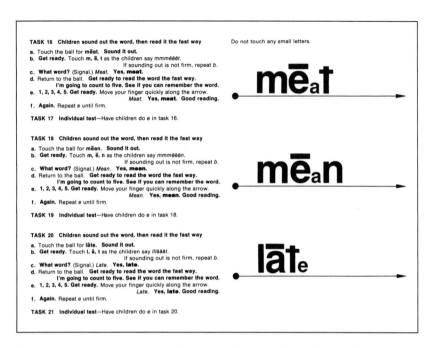

TASK 16 Children sound out the word, then read it the fast way   Do not touch any small letters.

a. Touch the ball for **mēat**. **Sound it out.**
b. **Get ready.** Touch m, ē, t as the children say *mmmēēēt*.
　　　　　　　　　　　　　　If sounding out is not firm, repeat *b*.
c. **What word?** (Signal.) *Meat*. **Yes, meat.**
d. Return to the ball. **Get ready to read the word the fast way.**
　　I'm going to count to five. See if you can remember the word.
e. **1, 2, 3, 4, 5. Get ready.** Move your finger quickly along the arrow.
　　　　　　　　　　　　　　Meat. **Yes, meat. Good reading.**
f. **Again.** Repeat *e* until firm.

TASK 17 **Individual test**—Have children do *e* in task 16.

TASK 18 Children sound out the word, then read it the fast way

a. Touch the ball for **mēan**. **Sound it out.**
b. **Get ready.** Touch m, ē, n as the children say *mmmēēēn*.
　　　　　　　　　　　　　　If sounding out is not firm, repeat *b*.
c. **What word?** (Signal.) *Mean*. **Yes, mean.**
d. Return to the ball. **Get ready to read the word the fast way.**
　　I'm going to count to five. See if you can remember the word.
e. **1, 2, 3, 4, 5. Get ready.** Move your finger quickly along the arrow.
　　　　　　　　　　　　　　Mean. **Yes, mean. Good reading.**
f. **Again.** Repeat *e* until firm.

TASK 19 **Individual test**—Have children do *e* in task 18.

TASK 20 Children sound out the word, then read it the fast way

a. Touch the ball for **lāte**. **Sound it out.**
b. **Get ready.** Touch l, ā, t as the children say *lllāāāt*.
　　　　　　　　　　　　　　If sounding out is not firm, repeat *b*.
c. **What word?** (Signal.) *Late*. **Yes, late.**
d. Return to the ball. **Get ready to read the word the fast way.**
　　I'm going to count to five. See if you can remember the word.
e. **1, 2, 3, 4, 5. Get ready.** Move your finger quickly along the arrow.
　　　　　　　　　　　　　　Late. **Yes, late. Good reading.**
f. **Again.** Repeat *e* until firm.

TASK 21 **Individual test**—Have children do *e* in task 20.

Teacher's Lesson Script from Reading Mastery I: Distar Reading *by Siegfried Engelmann and Elaine C. Bruner. (Reproduced with permission from Science Research Associates, Inc., Chicago, IL. Copyright 1983.)*

ing a heavy macron over letters representing long vowel sounds, printing consonant blends as joined letters, slightly changing the configuration of *d* to distinguish it from *b*, and omitting upper case formations except for *I*.

　　Comprehension activities at the prereading level include interpreting pictures and ordering events in sequence. At the reading level, comprehension skills are taught first in simple sentences and then in stories. In the early stages, children are asked to predict something about the content of pictures by first reading words related to the picture but presented on a preceding page. Once children are reading stories, oral comprehension questions, such as *wh* questions, are posed during the reading. In addition, the teacher summarizes the story and asks students to predict what will happen next.

　　In later stages, children answer written questions about the story. For explicit questions, the group is called upon to respond in unison, but for questions calling for divergent responses, such as giving opinions, individual response is requested. When students are able to read stories "the fast way" on first reading, each student's speed and accuracy are checked every fifth lesson. In addition, mastery tests are administered approximately every fifth lesson from the beginning of the program. Spelling instruction is optional in this program, though strongly encouraged. It is suggested that spelling be taught to the entire class if time does not allow small-group practice. The spelling curriculum follows the sequence of the reading curriculum. Spelling activities begin with children writing letters for dictated letter sounds and move on to their writing words and sentences. The Spelling Mastery program begins in second grade and continues through sixth-grade level. It starts with teaching basic phonemic spelling strategies and memorization of high-frequency irregular spellings, and later teaches morphographs (word parts that have meaning, such as the ending *tion*) and spelling rules.

Handwriting instruction is included in the reading curriculum and begins in Lesson 7 when children are first asked to write letter sounds (letter names are not yet introduced). Students are taught manuscript letter formations through tracing exercises with faded prompts (the amount of the model letters shown is gradually diminished). Minimal emphasis is placed on handwriting or on written expression in the DISTAR curriculum.

The recommended time for reading lessons is twenty-five to thirty minutes of group instruction, followed by fifteen to twenty minutes of independent work, five minutes of work check for each group, and ten minutes of group spelling practice. Students are given take-home assignments from the first day of the program.

Scheduling for DISTAR may vary among schools. In one inner-city school, for example, approximately 60 percent of the school day is allocated to DISTAR reading, math, and language in the first three grades, with one hour per subject area. (Meyer, Gersten, and Gutkin 1983).

TEACHER TRAINING

According to Becker (1977), a one-week preservice workshop, followed by one to two hours of inservice training a week (duration of period not specified) is usually adequate for teachers to learn DISTAR. Manuals are provided for trainers, just as scripts are provided for teachers. The training procedure involves demonstration, guided practice, and feedback. In the case of the schools that participated in Project Follow-Through, a project manager (university staff member) trained teachers individually or in groups (Meyer, Gersten, and Gutkin 1983). After initial training, skilled teachers often supervised apprentice teachers within the classroom (Becker 1977).

EVALUATION AND IMPLEMENTATION

DISTAR gained prominence as the only one of the nine instructional models in Project Follow-Through to effect significant gains in basic skills as compared to a traditional instructional approach (not described) that was administered to a control group of disadvantaged children. Pre- and posttests on the Wide Range Achievement Test indicated that DISTAR students had moved, on average, from the 18th to the 84th percentile in reading (word decoding) on national norms and from the 8th to the 49th percentile in spelling (Becker 1977). DISTAR students did not show the same degree of advantage in reading comprehension on the Metropolitan Achievement Test (MAT), averaging 10 percentile points below the national average, but they still scored significantly higher than students in the other model programs in this area. In both spelling and language, DISTAR students met the national average on the MAT.

A later study, conducted as a follow-up of original DISTAR participants from one inner-city school in New York, looked at the progress of nine cohorts (classes) of those students who had completed the first three levels of the program (Meyer, Gersten, and Gutkin 1983). It was found that DISTAR students continued to score at or above grade level on standardized reading tests in grades four and five, and that they scored notably above a comparison group of disadvantaged students from the same school district who had not received DISTAR instruction.

Tracing the progress of these same students into high school, Linda Meyer (1984) found that their advantage over the comparison group in reading persisted into ninth grade. Even more impressive was the finding that 34 percent of the DISTAR students had applied and been accepted to college, whereas only 18 percent of the non-DISTAR comparison students applied and 17 percent were accepted. Furthermore, the dropout rate for DISTAR students was almost half that for comparison subjects.

DISTAR is not without its detractors, however. A common criticism is that the scripted lessons place too much restriction on teachers. Becker (1977) counters this complaint with the argument that scripts increase teacher accountability and help supervisors track teacher and student progress. Elsa Bartlett (1979), in comparing DISTAR with the Open Court basal program, finds that DISTAR's modified orthography is particularly detrimental to disadvantaged children who find it difficult to make the transition to traditional orthography. Bartlett also maintains that DISTAR does not provide enough literacy enrichment. However, Isabel Beck and Ellen McCaslin (1978), in comparing eight reading programs on several dimensions, conclude that DISTAR is the best program for compensatory education.

Although DISTAR has been used with young elementary school students classified as learning disabled, some of whom may be dyslexic, research has not yet systematically investigated the effectiveness of the Reading Mastery program with this group of children. On the other hand, several studies have attempted to validate the success of the Direct Instruction remedial reading program, Corrective Reading, with older learning disabled children (see Chapter 19).

The implementation of the DISTAR model, as part of the federally funded Project Follow-Through may be unique, but it entailed several elements worth noting for school change policy making. The first important implementation feature, after the provision of funds, was the sponsorship of each Follow-Through program by the program developer, in DISTAR's case, the University of Oregon, and the assignment of a project manager to train the teachers and install each program. According to Linda Meyer, Russell Gersten, and Joan Gutkin (1983) who studied the implementation of DISTAR at P.S. 137 in New York City, the project manager spends up to forty days a year at the school, conducting inservice training and acting as coordinator between students, parents, faculty, and administration. The project manager is actively involved in setting up classroom schedules, monitoring teacher and student performance, and assigning students and staff. It would be helpful to know if having an external change agent serve as principal administrator rather than a local school official is relevant to the program's success.

An extremely imporant factor in the P.S. 137 program has been strong parental involvement and support from the start (Meyer, Gersten, and Gutkin 1983). In fact, parents were largely responsible for the school's selection as a Follow-Through site, as well as for the choice of the Direct Instruction Model. Despite budget cuts and high teacher turnover, parents in this school have apparently fought successfully to keep the DISTAR program in place for more than thirteen years since its origination.

Meyer, Gersten, and Gutkin (1983) assert that one of the major strengths of the DISTAR model that has promoted its longevity is the continuity and consistency from preservice to inservice training sessions to continuous classroom observation and demonstration. They cite the Rand Study (Berman and McLaughlin 1975) finding that hands-on technical assistance to teachers is crucial for bringing about educational change.

CHAPTER

10

Corrective Reading

BACKGROUND AND RATIONALE

Corrective Reading (Englemann et al. 1980) is an extension of Wesley Becker and Siegfried Englemann's Direct Instruction Model (DISTAR), developed for students in fourth through twelfth grades who have failed to achieve in other reading programs. Corrective Reading instruction is intended to compensate for a wide range of constitutional and environmental deficiencies that contribute to reading failure; these include mild mental retardation, neurological impairment, emotional disturbance, socio-economic deprivation, and language and cultural differences, as well as dyslexia or learning disabilities. Like DISTAR, the program is designed for group administration and is intended as a core rather than supplementary reading program; it has been used in both special and regular education settings.

CURRICULUM AND INSTRUCTION

The Corrective Reading curriculum is divided into two strands, Decoding and Comprehension, each having three levels of skill development (A, B, and C). Lessons are carefully arranged in sequence so that the skills taught are cumulative. Students are given a test covering both decoding and comprehension, to determine their placement in the program.

Specific lessons at each curriculum level serve as entry points. Students may be placed in one or both of the curriculum strands; if in both, they must be in the same or a lower comprehension than decoding level, because the sequence of reading vocabulary in the comprehension strand corresponds to that in the decoding program.

The objective of the decoding program, according to the Series Guide (Engelmann et al. 1980), is "to teach the skills required to accurately and fluently identify and pronounce words that appear in written passages." It should be pointed out, however, that the decoding strand also deals with reading comprehension; students are asked comprehension questions about passages they read orally.

Placement level in the decoding strand is determined by a student's speed and accuracy in reading a passage orally. Students not meeting baseline criteria are referred for DISTAR I instruction. Students with only minimal reading skills are placed in Level A: Word Attack Basics, which contains sixty lessons. The major instructional goal at this level is to teach the idea that most words are regularly spelled and can be read by blending the letter sounds. Individual letter sounds are taught, first in isolation and then in words. Words are read first in isolation and then in unrelated sentences to avoid predictable context and discourage guessing, the latter strategy being the one most of these students have relied on unsuccessfully to compensate for their lack of letter-sound knowledge.

Only the most commonly used sound for each letter symbol is introduced at this level. This is the stated rationale for teaching the short sound for the vowel *a* and the long sound for the vowel *e* in Lesson 1. Not until Lesson 23 is the short *e* sound introduced; long *a* is not presented until Level B. The digraph *ee* is presented at the same time as the open syllable for long *e* (as in "me") to demonstrate /e/. This practice represents the principle of instructional economy whereby strategies and rules are kept as simple as possible (Gersten, Woodward, and Darch 1986). For this reason too, terms such as "vowels," "double consonants," or "final *e* words" are avoided. The long sound for *o* as it appears in the digraphs *ol* and *or* is taught as well as short *o* in Level A, whereas only the short sounds for *u* and *i* are introduced at this level. Practice in discriminating vowel sounds is provided by having students identify medial sounds in one-syllable words, for example, "Which word has the middle sound ăăăă: bean, ban, ben?"

As in DISTAR, pronunciation of letters and words is practiced by first sounding them out slowly and then saying them fast. When irregular words are first introduced in Lesson 46, the distinction is made between how they are spelled and how they are said. Students first sound out the words, pronouncing and blending the individual letter sounds, for example wwwăăăsss for "was." Then the teacher gives the correct pronunciation ("wuz").

According to the program's authors, 60 to 80 percent of Corrective Reading students enter at Level B: Decoding Strategies, which comprises 140 lessons. The focus of the curriculum at this level is on long and short vowels, vowel-consonant digraphs, vowel digraphs, diphthongs, and common word endings. Long-short vowel confusion errors are referred to as "same vowel mistakes," and teachers are given specific instructions for correcting these errors. Students are asked to note the presence or absence of a final *e* in the word missed which indicates the pronunciation of the preceding vowel. After pronouncing the word correctly, the students repeat the word. The teacher then writes the word as the students mistakenly pronounced it and has them read it. She changes it back to its correct spelling and asks the students to read it again. This model-test-discriminate-retest approach is used as a correcting procedure throughout the program. For correcting vowel confusion errors in words with endings (e.g., "robe" for "robber"), the teacher underlines the word from the beginning to the second letter after the vowel (robber), and students are told, "If the last letter of the underlined part is *e* or *i,* you hear a letter name in the word" (Engelmann et al. 1978). Phonic rules are not taught as spelling rules in Corrective Reading as they are in most remedial approaches. Although Level A includes spelling dictation exercises, the Corrective Reading curriculum includes little direct spelling instruction. Two types of word reading exercises are provided at Level B: similar list presentation, which emphasizes orthographic differences between words that share features (e.g., hat, hate, hated) and random list presentation of unrelated words which requires remembering specific features of words.

In addition to word attack exercises, Level B involves group story reading which uses a round robin format, each student reading a sentence or two. Stories contain words introduced in the lessons. Oral reading errors are corrected on the spot, and the student is asked to reread the sentence. The teacher asks comprehension questions during the story reading, calling on individual students to answer. The questions not only ensure that all students are following the text, but also provide a story grammar framework for comprehending its contents, for example: Who is the story about? What does he or she want to do? What happens when he or she tries to do it? What happens in the end? According to Russell Gersten, John Woodward, and Craig Darch (1986), who are strong proponents of Corrective Reading, students begin to "internalize these four questions and generalize this framework to other narrative material." From Lesson 81 on, students are asked to write answers to additional comprehension questions after the story has been read.

Oral reading checks are conducted at the end of each lesson in Level B. Students read aloud individually the same 100-word passage from the story read in that lesson, as well as a second 100-word passage from the previous lesson. Selected peers may act as checkers, according to the pro-

Lesson 108

WORD-ATTACK SKILLS

Individual turns

After presenting each of the following exercises to the group, call on individual students. Each student should read one word or more. Present words that were difficult for the group.

EXERCISE 1 Sound combination: oi
1. Print in a column on the board: **oil, voice, spoil, hoist, foiled, moist, joined.** Underline as indicated.
2. Point to **oi** in **oil**.
   What sound? Touch. *oy*
   Point to **oil**.
   What word? Signal. *Oil.*
3. Repeat step 2 for **voice, spoil.**
4. For each remaining word:
   Point to the word. Pause. **What word?** Signal.
5. Repeat the list until firm.

EXERCISE 2 Endings buildups
1. Print on the board: **heat, splash, boil, clamp.**
2. For each word:
   Point to the word. Pause. **What word?** Signal.
3. Change the words to **heater, splasher, boiler, clamper.** Repeat step 2.
4. Change the words to **heats, splashes, boils, clamps.** Repeat step 2.
5. Change the words to **heated, splashed, boiled, clamped.** Repeat step 2.
6. Repeat steps 1–5 until firm.
7. Change the words to **heater, splashes, boils, clamped.** Repeat step 2.
8. Repeat the exercise until firm.

EXERCISE 3 Word practice
1. Print on the board: **batch, scare, recall, invisible, upstairs, couch, watched, stinky, mirror, cracked, shelf, chairs, else, easy, spun, basement, quickly, Herman, slowly, Fern, women.**
2. For each word:
   Point to the word. Pause. **What word?** Signal.
3. Repeat the list until firm.

EXERCISE 4 Word conversions
1. Print on the board the words that are not in brackets:

fell [feel]	call [carl]	poach [pouch]
boiling [bailing]	tool [toil]	coach [crouch]
coach [couch]	malt [melt]	pond [pound]
beet [belt]	want [went]	clod [cloud]

2. For each word:
   Point to the word. Pause. **What word?** Signal.
3. Change each word to the word in brackets next to it. Then repeat step 2.
4. Convert each word back to its original form. Repeat steps until firm.

EXERCISE 5 Word practice on worksheet
1. Pass out the worksheet for lesson 108.
2. **Point to the underlined part of the first word.** Check.
   What sound? Signal. *ar.*
   What word? Signal. *Lark.*
3. For each word with an underlined part:
   Next word. Check.
   What sound? Signal.
   What word? Signal.
4. For each word that does not have an underlined part:
   Next word. Check.
   What word? Signal.
5. Repeat each row of words until firm.

GROUP READING

EXERCISE 6 Story reading
1. **Everybody, touch the story.** Check.
2. **The error limit for this story is twelve. If the group reads the story with twelve errors or less, you can earn up to 10 points.**
3. Call on a student to read the title.
   What do you think this story is about?
4. Call on individual students to each read one or two sentences.
5. Ask the comprehension questions below during the story reading. The numbers in the story indicate at what point each question should be asked. Call on individual students to answer each question.
   1. **In what ways was Irma going to have fun with the paint?**
   2. **Where did Irma rub the paint?**
   3. **Where didn't Irma rub the paint? How would her eyes have spoiled the trick? How did Irma make her eyes look invisible?**
   4. **What is the only part of Irma that is not invisible? What kind of hand is Irma going to give her boarders?**
   5. **What are the boarders doing? What is the woman on TV doing?**
   6. **Why is Irma talking in a loud voice?**
   7. **What did Irma's boarders do when they saw the hand?**
6. Award points quickly.
7. If the group makes more than twelve errors, tell them they earn no points for the story reading. Then do one of the following:
   a. If time allows, repeat the story reading immediately. If the group now succeeds, complete the lesson (individual checkouts) and do the next lesson the following day.
   b. If there isn't time to repeat the story reading, tell the group they will have to repeat the story the following day.
8. Point to the written comprehension questions.
   Remember: write the answers to the questions while the others are being checked out.

CHECKOUTS

EXERCISE 7 Individual reading checkouts
1. Each student reads to the checker:
   a. A 100-word passage from story 108 as the first reading of this lesson.
   b. A 100-word passage from story 107 as the second reading.
   Those who make no errors on the first reading automatically receive 5 points credit for the second reading. They do not do a second reading.
2. Each student records points in box C of the point chart.

EXERCISE 8 Written questions checkout
1. Call on individual students to answer each question. Remind the students to mark each incorrect answer.
2. **Answer key: 1.** He wanted Irma to help move the couch. **2.** She rubbed paint on a pair of sun glasses. **3.** Her right hand **4.** "Uh, buh, duh, buh, buh, uh."
3. Remind the students to record the points they earned on their charts.

END OF LESSON 108

Teacher's Lesson Script from Corrective Reading Series Guide *by Siegfried Engelmann, Wesley C. Becker, Susan Hanner, and Gary Johnson. (Reproduced with permission from Science Research Associates, Inc., Chicago, IL. Copyright 1978.)*

gram's authors, but most studies of Corrective Reading application report the use of teacher aides for this purpose. Every fifth lesson requires a timed reading check, so that a record of speed as well as accuracy can be kept for each student.

Level C: Skills Applications comprises 140 lessons. This top level of the decoding strand continues instruction in word attack skills, reviewing previously introduced digraphs, diphthongs, less common phonemes and syllables, and teaching new ones. It introduces some of the more common affixes. Exercises for teaching these elements follow the formats used in the lower curriculum levels.

Preparing students to read textbook material is a major objective of the Level C: Decoding curriculum. Toward this end more than 600 new vocabulary words are introduced, defined, and presented in text. The basis for selecting these words, however, is not explained; the selections seem to vary widely in frequency rating: "prevented," for example, as compared to "prestidigitator." An effort is made to expose students to "sentence types and conventions that characterize text material" (Englemann et al. 1980), such as the passive voice. Group story reading at this level requires answering both literal and inferential comprehension questions in writing. In addition, students read nonfiction information passages during individual oral reading checks. After Lesson 70 they also read together magazine and newpaper articles on topics of their choice.

The program's authors maintain that students who complete Level C are "fluent decoders who make only occasional decoding errors when reading materials that contain a fairly broad vocabulary and a variety of sentence types" (Englemann et al. 1980). The authors believe that although students may still have comprehension deficits which limit their overall reading ability, their decoding problems at this point are essentially remediated.

Although reading is involved, Corrective Reading's comprehension strand is devoted primarily to the development of cognitive skills and language skills that relate to academic work. Level A, called Thinking Basics, is geared to students who lack essential concepts underlying school curriculum content, who may also have a limited store of background information for processing school material and may also manifest difficulty repeating orally presented information. Each lesson has three segments. The first, Thinking Operations, teaches the following concepts which are relevant to content area material: analogies and/or basic evidence, classification, deductions, definitions, description, inductions, opposites, same, statement inference, and true–false. These are taught directly by the teacher to the group, through example and repetition. In the second lesson segment, students apply these concepts in workbook exercises. In the third, the Information track, they are taught calendar facts (months, seasons, holidays) and biology facts (animals and their classifications); additionally, they learn to recite short poems.

While somewhat more advanced than Level A students, those entering Level B: Comprehension Skills may still lack basic information, such as calendar facts. The major thrust at this level is "to teach and reinforce a substantial amount of information and many operations" (Engelmann et al. 1980). Areas covered in this curriculum include: Reasoning Skills (deductions, basic evidence, analogies, contradictions, and similes); Information Skills (classification, body systems, body rules, and economic rules); Vocabulary Skills (definitions); Sentence Skills (parts of speech, subject/predicate, sentence combinations, and sentence analysis); Comprehension Skills (inference and following directions); and Writing Skills (writing directions, editing, writing paragraphs, and writing stories). Each lesson involves group oral work, oral workbook exercises, and independent workbook exercises. Students check each others' answers to these exercises.

At Level C: Concept Applications, the instructional emphasis is on teaching students to apply independently the skills they have learned. Five categories of application skills are taught in this curriculum: Organizing Information (main idea, outlining, specific-general, morals, and visual-spatial information); Operating On Information (deductions, basic evidence, argument rules, ought statements, and contradictions); Using Sources of Information (basic comprehension passages, words or deductions, maps, pictures and graphs, and supporting evidence); Communicating Information (definitions, combining sentences, editing, and getting meaning from context); and Using Information (writing directions, filling out forms, and identifying contradictory directions). The first two operational categories are classified as "higher-order skills" and the last three as "basic tools." A major change in instructional procedure takes place at Level C—rather than the teacher's presenting scripted lessons, students read the lesson scripts in their workbooks. The teacher monitors their processing of the workbook exercises, asking questions to ensure understanding. Increasing demands are placed on writing performance at this level.

All Corrective Reading lessons are designed to be administered daily in thirty-five to forty minute periods, although several effectiveness studies report somewhat longer periods and often more than one period per day. A lesson is designed to be covered within a single period but may be repeated if mastery is not attained by all students in the class. Individual mastery checks, as well as the monitoring of group responses, provide ongoing information on student performance and allow for repetition or acceleration of lessons if needed.

A point system serves as a behavior management device at all curriculum levels. Students are awarded points for successful performance in both group and individual activities throughout the Corrective Reading curriculum; a point schedule is provided for each lesson. In group activities, all students must meet performance criteria in order for any points to be awarded. Bonus points may be given for success or persistence on especially difficult activities or to encourage positive behaviors, such as being on time for lessons. Students keep records of points earned. Weekly summaries of accumulated points are intended to provide positive feedback to further reinforce student learning.

Behavior management also entails having each student who enters the program sign a contract indicating his or her willingness to cooperate and work hard. The teacher explains the point system, the need for daily class attendance, and the penalty for making negative comments about peers. The penalty for making fun of another student is paid by the group as a whole to further discourage this detrimental behavior.

As in DISTAR, the hallmark of Corrective Reading is its unique approach to direct group instruction. All lessons are scripted; teachers are told exactly what to say and do. All student exercises are presented in formats; similar activities follow the same formats, which simplifies the teacher's task and serves as a prompt for students to apply a learned skill to new examples. Correction procedures, both general and specific, are carefully spelled out for all activities. Hand signals are used by teachers to direct student response in unison. These allow for fast paced instruction, which is believed to help sustain student attention, increase student achievement, and reduce auditory memory demands on students. The signals include: the hand-drop, which indicates that students should respond in unison in naming items pointed to on the chalkboard or in their workbooks; the audible signal (clapping, finger snapping, foot tapping) to redirect student attention; the sound-out signal (the teacher runs her finger along a line under the letter or word to be pronounced), which controls the pace of blending letter sounds; and the sequential-response signal (the teacher holds up one finger to call for a first response and then two fingers to signal a second response), as when students are asked to name two important facts in a story.

The materials used in Corrective Reading Instruction include: the Series Guide which provides an overview of the entire program; a teacher's manual for each level of a curriculum strand, which provides a curriculum guide for that level and the presentation scripts for each lesson; a student workbook which contains stories to be read and/or exercises to be carried out; and, at Level C, a student textbook which contains the lesson scripts to be read by the students themselves.

TEACHER TRAINING

Teacher preparation for Corrective Reading has not been formalized as in some other remedial programs and may vary with schools and school districts, depending upon their requirements and their budgets. However, training can be arranged through The Association for Direct Instruction (see Resource and Teacher Training Guide in Appendix). On the East Coast it is provided by the Center for Direct Instruction which is based in New York City. This training is usually conducted in one six-hour session, most often in a school, though sometimes in university sponsored workshops offering graduate credit. Follow-up on-site supervision in classrooms or further consultation to schools is available for an additional fee.

Reporting on the implementation of Corrective Reading with learning disabled and mildly retarded adolescents in a rural/suburban school district, Edward Polloway and Michael Epstein (1986) indicate that teacher preparation involved two full days of inservice training. The first session provided an overview of the program and the instructional methodology, as well as information about placement testing, grouping, and scheduling. The second session focused specifically on teaching techniques. However, even with two training sessions, considerable variability in teacher competence was noted during program implementation.

In a model demonstration project using DISTAR, described by Michael Epstein and Douglas Cullinan (1981), teachers received three to four days of training from university personnel before program implementation. In addition, they were observed once a week in their classrooms by project staff members throughout the school year. Russell Gersten, John Woodward, and Craig Darch (1986) caution that teacher competence with Direct Instruction is not assured, despite the provision of scripted lessons. Based on their own experience in implementing Direct Instruction programs, these researchers maintain that teachers benefit most from training that takes place in the actual classroom and involves the specific application of teaching techniques first modeled by the trainer.

Epstein and Cullinan employed teacher aides in their implementation of Corrective Reading. The aides were trained directly in the classroom and received weekly follow-up supervision alongside the classroom teachers. Cynthia Herr (1984) has found teacher aides to be extremely useful for monitoring oral reading checks and supervising work with adult students in Corrective Reading classes.

EVALUATION AND IMPLEMENTATION

Studies have investigated the use of Corrective Reading with students having a range of mild handicapping conditions, as well as with students for whom English is a second language (Polloway and Epstein 1986). Several of these studies have examined the program's effectiveness with students classified as learning disabled. Polloway and Epstein (1986), for example, measured the effectiveness of Corrective Reading with a mixed group of educable mentally retarded (EMR) and learning disabled (LD) sixth- through twelfth-grade students by comparing reading gains achieved over a year of Corrective Reading instruction to gains made in the previous year of special education instruction. Using the Peabody Individual Achievement Test (PIAT), they found significantly greater gains after Corrective Reading instruction than in the previous year for EMR as well as LD subjects, in both word recognition and reading comprehension. Although the LD subjects had greater gains than the EMR subjects on word recognition scores, no significant differences were found in reading comprehension gain scores between the two subject types. However, Polloway and Epstein suggest that the latter finding may be due to the failure of the PIAT to tap the comprehension skills taught in Corrective Reading. In support of this suggestion, they cite teachers' claims that the PIAT underestimates student achievement in this area.

Epstein and Cullinan (1981) investigated the effects of a federally funded model implementation of Corrective Reading with nine-year-old students classified as learning disabled. (It is worth noting that their Slosson IQ scores ranged only from 76 to 86.) Subjects were randomly assigned to self-contained classrooms, two of which used Corrective Reading. The other classroom used unspecified remedial procedures and served as the control condition. At the end of one school year, reading scores (posttest only) were higher for both groups receiving Corrective Reading than the comparison group. However, John Lloyd along with Epstein and Cullinan, in reporting on the same study, acknowledge that neither of the experimental groups reached normal reading achievement levels in that year and suggest that more instructional time is needed to reach such a goal (Lloyd, Epstein, and Cullinan 1981). It should also be mentioned that the number of subjects in each group was low (seven to eight), as was the case in the Polloway and Epstein study (four to eight). Though optimal for instructional purposes, such small samples weaken the validity of the outcome analyses.

In terms of progam implementation, Epstein and Cullinan (1981) maintain that although the planning, training, and evaluation costs of Corrective Reading are considerably higher than the cost of most basal reading programs, the expense is on par with that of other learning disability programs. A greater challenge, but one worth meeting they believe, is convincing school personnel of the need for carefully supervised, highly structured, task-oriented direct instruction with learning disabled children.

CHAPTER

Project READ (Calfee)

BACKGROUND AND RATIONALE

Project READ was developed by Robert Calfee and his associates at Stanford University, in collaboration with several elementary schools in the Palo Alto area of California. It was initiated in 1981 in one school with a broad-based assessment of the reading curriculum then in place, followed by a five-day teacher workshop to assess the curriculum needs. This led to the creation of a teacher's manual, *THE BOOK: Components of Reading Instruction* (Calfee and Associates 1981–1984), which serves as the curriculum guide for Project READ.

The manual is based upon the contention that the academic curriculum in most schools today lacks coherence. Calfee and his colleague, Marcia Henry maintain that the content of school subject matter and materials are fragmented; that teachers are not provided an explicit conceptual framework for teaching; and that the principal no longer plays the originally intended role of "principal teacher." Project READ seeks to remedy these deficiencies by providing a "parsimonious and coherent theoretical framework for representing the various elements that comprise a reading program" (Calfee and Henry 1985). Although the program was developed for conventional classroom use in elementary schools, its authors feel its basic assumptions apply to all learners and, thus, that it should benefit students at risk for reading failure, as well as those who show normal potential.

179

Calfee and Henry (1985) distinguish two kinds of learning: "learn-ing-by-doing" and "learning-by-knowing." The former, which may oc-cur in any environment, is experiential and incremental. The latter, which results from formal education, tends to be all or nothing. Stressing the need to teach children how to learn by knowing, Calfee and Henry state:

> A major goal of schooling is to transmit to the student the most significant facets of our cultural heritage, knowledge that is most efficiently trans-ferred through learning-by-knowing. In addition, the school teaches the student how to acquire knowledge in this fashion (learning to learn, if you will, of a special variety). (Calfee and Henry 1985, p. 145)

THE BOOK emphasizes four instructional propositions, the first being *simplicity:* complex tasks should be broken down into a "small num-ber of relatively coherent subtasks." The second is that language skills (reading, writing, speaking, and even listening) are *interrelated* and should be taught as such. The third proposition is that teaching the *formal use of language* is one of the most important goals of schooling. The fourth prop-osition is that *direct teaching,* combined with *small-group discussion,* is an es-sential component of effective reading instruction.

CURRICULUM AND INSTRUCTION

The basic curriculum components of Project READ are decoding, vocabulary, sentence and paragraph comprehension, and text comprehen-sion. Critical to the program's philosophy of coherence and parsimony is the fact that any lesson should focus on only one of these curriculum areas. For expediency, the program is adaptable to any basal reader series cur-rently in use. Any or all of the four curriculum areas can be applied to a particular basal reader selection, but only one at a time.

The instructional format for any lesson consists of four parts: the opening (introduction and stated goal of the lesson); the middle activity (discussion, question asking, problem solving, summarizing, recording results); closing (review of what was accomplished in lesson—usually conducted by the teacher); and follow-up activities (practice and reinforce-ment of skills learned). Teachers are urged to develop a script for each lesson that follow this four-part format; model scripts are provided in *THE BOOK.*

An especially notable aspect of the decoding curriculum is the at-tention given to etymology. In teaching word attack strategies, a major distinction is made between words of Anglo-Saxon origin, which are taught first, and words of Romance origin, which are introduced later. *THE BOOK* discusses the differences between these two etymological strands and provides teachers with a good background of the English language, a missing element in most teacher preparation programs. Words of Greek origin, which are largely scientific or technical words, are recognized as a third etymological strand.

The two basic distinguishing characteristics brought forth about Anglo-Saxon words are the fact that they are shorter and that they comprise more letter-sounds than there are letters in the alphabet. These sounds are represented either by digraphs or by markers, such as final silent-*e*. Romance words, by comparison, are longer and more complex. The long and short vowel markings in these words are less consistent, and there are likely to be unstressed schwa syllables. Vowel digraphs in Romance words, on the other hand, are less common and more regular.

THE BOOK essentially provides a framework for teaching word attack skills and spelling strategies, rather than detailed instructions. Conspicuously absent is the term "phonics." Calfee states that there is as yet no known best way to teach decoding skills and seems to leave the choice of instructional method up to teachers. However, the scripts provided follow an analytic approach.

Decoding instruction progresses sequentially from regular short words and the basic spelling patterns (short vowel patterns, long vowel patterns, vowel digraphs having one or two sounds, etc.) to compound words to polysyllabic words. Common sight words ("weirdo words"), which must be memorized, are introduced early. Calfee believes that decoding instruction should not be dropped altogether in later grades, because many students have trouble reading longer polysyllabic words. The emphasis at this point should be placed on structural analysis, as well as on developing an awareness of word origins.

Believing that vocabulary is best taught within conceptual frameworks, Calfee has incorporated two innovative instructional techniques that he refers to as "webbing" and "weaving." Webbing involves teaching each new word within a set of words that are semantically related, as opposed to presenting them in unrelated word lists. In the webbing script the teacher selects a target word or concept and tells the students to generate related words. These words are then arranged by the class into categories, and a webbing diagram is drawn up.

The weaving script begins with a group of words, selected by the teacher, which are then discussed by the class and organized as conceptual structures, either hierarchical semantic networks or matrixes. In addition to structuring, numerous alternative activities can be included in the weaving script, for example, finding evidence, making comparisons, hypothesizing relationships. Calfee suggests that a weaving lesson can provide preparation for writing an expository passage.

Building morphological knowledge is an important aspect of effective vocabulary instruction, according to Calfee, particularly at the secondary level. He advocates teaching the recognition and meaning of

```
SCRIPT:  Webbing
                       AIM:  To make students aware of how words are related
   STUDENTS' PREREQUISITES:  Knowledge of basic meanings of target words
     TEACHER'S PREPARATION:  Select target word
                             Choose categories for web


OPENING              ┌─────────────────────────────────────────────────────┐
                     │ Today we're going to study about how words are related│
                     │ so we can get a better understanding of what a word   │
                     │ means.                                                │
                     │                                                       │
                     │ (Explain the concept of a web)                        │
                     │                                                       │
                     │ Today we're going to work with the word _____   │
                     └─────────────────────────────────────────────────────┘

MODAL                ┌─────────────────────────────────────────────────────┐
MIDDLE ACTIVITY      │ What are some of the things the word _____ (write on│
                     │ board) makes you think of?                            │
   FREE GENERATION   │ Let's go around the room, each of you tell me what you │
                     │ think of when you hear _____. Let's see if everyone   │
                     │ can give a different answer.                          │
                     │                                                       │
                     │ I'll write on the board what you say, and we'll try to │
                     │ organize your answers.                                │
                     │                                                       │
                     │ (Write responses in a webbing plan as illustrated in  │
                     │ Blackboard Examples . . . then:)                      │
     Categorization  │ Look how the words are arranged.                      │
                     │ Why do you think I put certain words together?        │
                     │ Why are . . . (e.g., fur, black nose, pointed         │
                     │ ears together?)                                       │
                     │ Why are . . . (e.g., bark, bite, run together?)       │
                     │                                                       │
                     │ Can you think of any other words to add to the web?   │
                     └─────────────────────────────────────────────────────┘

CLOSING              ┌─────────────────────────────────────────────────────┐
                     │ What have we learned about the word _____?           │
                     │                                                       │
                     │ What are some of the categories we used to organize   │
                     │ our web?                                              │
                     │                                                       │
                     │ Why did we put certain words in the same category?    │
                     │                                                       │
                     │ How did webbing help us understand word meanings?     │
                     └─────────────────────────────────────────────────────┘

THE BOOK
Calfee/Stanford  81/83a                                          Vocabulary
```

Teacher's Lesson Script from The Book *by Robert Calfee and Associates, 1981–1984, School of Education, Stanford University, Palo Alto, CA. (Reproduced with permission from the author.)*

morphological elements by first presenting concrete examples and only later introducing the rules. This places responsibility on teachers to acquire more than the rudimentary linguistic knowledge provided in most teacher preparation programs.

Although Calfee cites sentence and paragraph comprehension as one of the four basic instructional components of Project READ, the current version of *THE BOOK* contains no directions for teaching sentence or paragraph structure, nor any mention of syntax or grammar. Comprehension instruction begins at the text level, where a major distinction is made between narrative and expository structure. Students are first taught to recognize the various elements of story structure, such as time and setting, characters, sequence of events, and main theme. Activities (for example, creating graphs to depict the events in a story or making outlines to describe the episodes) are intended to lead to an awareness of these elements.

Calfee points out that most children come to school with a basic knowledge of story structure and that basal reader material in the early grades is almost exclusively narrative. In contrast, they receive little exposure to exposition in these grades and they are rarely provided with a knowledge of expository structure. *THE BOOK* provides a classification of expository styles, focusing on two basic catagories: description and sequence. Suggested teaching activities are much the same as those for narration, for example, discussing the structure and purpose of the text, making outlines, locating and labeling topic sentences, diagramming.

Writing instruction is not dealt with in *THE BOOK,* although Calfee states that composition and comprehension go hand in hand; his suggestions for reading comprehension activities does include writing. Spelling is taught concomitantly with decoding.

Project READ teaches test-taking strategies as well. Instruction in this area also involves the use of scripts and provides a conceptual framework by incorporating webbing activities into the scripts.

TEACHER TRAINING

Training for Project READ teachers involves a three day workshop. The workshop has four major objectives: (1) to familiarize teachers with the program's theoretical foundations; (2) to enable teachers to evaluate instructional materials from the basal reader series used in their schools within this theoretical framework; (3) to demonstrate the use of instructional scripts; and (4) to demonstrate small-group problem solving as an instructional approach.

In the fall, following the workshop, staff members visit the target schools to demonstrate sample scripts and to help teachers apply the project's principles. The newly trained teachers are observed as they try out scripts in their classrooms. For additional support, two or three day-long follow-up sessions are held in each school for progress evaluation and further instruction as needed. All Project READ teachers are interviewed at the end of the school year to determine their overall impressions of the program and their success in implementing the program's philosophy. Monthly newsletters are circulated to provide a network of up-to-date information on program development.

EVALUATION AND IMPLEMENTATION

So far, Project READ has been established in over a dozen schools in California. Its authors report that in these schools standardized test scores have increased by one-half to one full grade level equivalent (Calfee, Henry, and Funderburg 1988). The authors claim that the quantity and quality of student writing has been enhanced.

Informal evaluation procedures, based on observation and interviews, indicate improvement in teacher attitudes, morale, and self-confidence, as well as in teacher competence. In addition, teachers report a closer professional relationship with other faculty members (Calfee and Henry 1985). Parents and students are generally enthusiastic about the program. The most difficult skill for teachers to learn apparently is the development of scripts; it was found that additional preparation time and ongoing support was needed for this purpose in the first year.

Calfee and his associates have drawn several conclusions concerning the implementation of educational change in schools. Their first tenet is that any change must be initiated and sustained at the local school level (Calfee, Henry, and Funderburg 1988). A second premise, which has extensive empirical backing, is that the school principal must assume a strong leadership role. Before working with a school, Calfee and his colleagues make sure that they can count on the principal's support and even insist that the principal participate in the project's training program. Another condition, which they consider essential for effective reading instruction, is the creation of a common conceptual framework for this instruction. Too often, they maintain, new programs focus only on a single aspect of reading, which further fragments the existing reading curriculum.

The question of whether or not the instruction provided in Project READ is either appropriate or adequate for dyslexic students must now be addressed. Although the program's conceptual framework might have value for teachers working with reading disabled students, these students may require a greater degree of explicit instruction in the various skill areas than is offered by the program as it is now written, particularly in decoding. In addition, it is likely that they will need considerably more instructional time to master these skills.

Recently, Marcia Henry (1987) conducted a study with school-classified learning disabled students in grades three through five in which she combined Orton-Gillingham instruction with the Project READ approach, calling the revised curriculum Project READ PLUS. Although a strong advocate of the Orton-Gillingham principles, Henry believes that reading disabled students, as well as normally achieving students, need more exposure to syllable and morphemic patterns than is provided in the Orton-Gillingham approach or is generally provided in basal reader programs. She maintains that in reading unfamiliar words, proficient readers first look for meaningful morphemic patterns, then for syllable patterns, and only if these strategies fail, focus on letter-sound associations. Henry also believes that all students will benefit from a greater knowledge of etymology. She therefore has reorganized and expanded the Orton-Gillingham curriculum to incorporate the four instructional components of Project READ: letter–sound correspondences, syllable patterns, morphemic patterns, and word origins, the last component taking into account the three major etymological strands of the English language, Anglo–Saxon, Romance, and Greek. The revised curriculum also teaches a technical vocabulary which allows students to talk about decoding concepts. This vocabulary includes words such as "grapheme," "phoneme," "consonant digraph," and "schwa."

A primary goal of the Project READ PLUS curriculum is to develop metalinguistic and metacognitive awareness among students, to encourage them to reflect upon and monitor their reading and writing. Instruction in Henry's study took place in small group settings and involved extensive discussion among students and teacher about decoding concepts and strategies. Unfortunately, because the study did not include a comparison group of disabled readers who were not given Project READ PLUS instruction, a valid evaluation of the effects of Project READ PLUS with disabled readers was not possible. The learning disabled subjects did not learn as much as a group of normally achieving students also receiving Project READ PLUS instruction, and they seemed to need more time to master the decoding terminology and concepts. Nevertheless, Henry observed pre-to-posttest gains among the learning disabled subjects on all the decoding subskills that were tested and, in addition, found that they enjoyed discussing how to decode and spell words.

CHAPTER

Writing to Read

W riting to Read was designed as a beginning reading program for children in the educational mainstream rather than as a remedial program for dyslexic children; however, I am describing the program in this book because it embodies many of the instructional principles so important for dyslexic children. These include an emphasis on teaching letter-sound correspondences and mastery of the alphabetic principle, the built-in promotion of phonological awareness, the incorporation of multi-sensory activities, and the opportunity for extensive practice or overlearning. Furthermore, I believe two additional aspects of this recently developed program may have potential for dyslexic children: (1) a systematic methodology for teaching beginning reading and spelling skills through writing, and (2) the innovative application of computer technology for teaching these skills.

BACKGROUND AND RATIONALE

Writing to Read was created by John Henry Martin, a retired school superintendent with thirty-five years of experience as an educator. He defines Writing to Read as a "computer-based instructional system designed to develop writing and reading skills of kindergarten and first grade children" (Martin and Friedberg 1986). The program was developed in cooperation with International Business Machines Corporation (IBM). It was piloted over a five-year period with nearly 1,000 children and was subjected to a nationwide evaluation from 1981 to 1984 with over 10,000 children in 105 schools within twenty-two school districts in metropolitan, suburban, and rural settings.

The rationale for Writing to Read derives from the theories of Maria Montessori (1964), Carol Chomsky (1979), and other educators who have proposed that young children more easily learn to read words that they themselves have composed, using the language they have acquired, than they learn to read words written by someone else in language that may be less familiar. (See Chapter 4, The Reading-Writing Relationship.) In their book, *Writing to Read,* which describes the program, Martin and his co-author, Ardy Friedberg, state that most normal children enter school knowing more than 2,000 words that they are able to use in a sophisticated syntax "nearly as complex as that used by adults" (Martin and Friedberg 1986). They can readily apply this knowledge to writing the letter sounds of English in words, sentences, and stories, which will lead them to grasp the alphabetic principle in a very short time. Writing to Read, according to Martin, teaches the alphabetic principle and phonemic spelling, while utilizing the educational potential of the computer and the electric typewriter, in combination with multisensory stimulation. Martin has called this a process approach, as compared to a basal reader method in which the vocabulary is controlled.

CURRICULUM AND INSTRUCTION

Despite Martin's definition of Writing to Read as a computer-based instructional system, the computer is only one of six different "work stations" in which the curriculum is conducted. Students spend a maximum of only fifteen minutes a day at the Computer Station. The other stations are Writing/Typing, Work Journal, Listening Library, Multi-Sensory, and Make Words. Materials used in the program include IBM PC jr Personal Computers, IBM Selectric typewriters, cassette tape players, prerecorded audio cassettes, audio headphones, classic childrens' books, Writing to Read work journals, writing utensils (soft lead pencils, chalk) and various multisensory materials, such as sand trays and clay. For much of the curriculum, students work in pairs.

Instruction begins at the Computer Station where ten cycles of three words each are taught. Forty-two phonemes are introduced sound by sound within the context of these words. Macrons are used to indicate long vowel sounds. Directions are presented to students via audio cassettes. In each exercise students work on only one of the three words in each cycle.

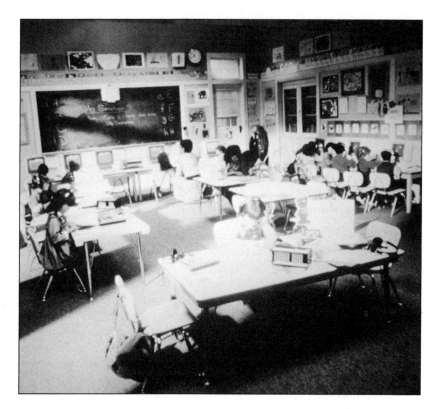

A Writing to Read *Center. (Photograph reproduced with permission from IBM Corporation.)*

The daily lesson begins with the student or students selecting one of the three words that appear in a list on the screen. If, for example, the word is "pig," the picture of the animal appears in the center of the screen and the letters of the word appear at the periphery. The voice on the cassette introduces the word and asks the student to say the word while the word flashes on the screen. Next the voice introduces the initial sound, /p/, and asks the student to say it and type it. As each letter is typed, it moves to its proper position in the word in the center of the screen. The spelling procedure is then repeated without the provision of the whole word on the screen. The third exercise requires the student to say each letter sound in rhythm while clapping his hands and then while stamping his feet. After the student has studied all three words in this manner, he goes on to the mastery test on which he is asked to type each of the three words. If two mistakes are made or too much time spent, the system reverts back to the lesson and the child resumes the initial tasks until he realizes where his mistake lies, at which point he can revert to the mastery test and correct his error.

The treatment of errors in the computer program comprises two important principles. First, correct responses are accepted at all times, even if typed prematurely; letters are stored in memory until the appropriate time for their inclusion. Second, incorrect responses are not accepted; if they are not self-corrected, the correct letters flash from the periphery of the screen.

The accumulating phonemes in words taught are positioned on the periphery. In this way,

> A child learns first subliminally, then slowly more concretely and consciously, that letters operate as visible symbols of the sounds of spoken words and that the twenty-six letters in various combinations can make all the words they can speak. (Martin and Friedberg 1986)

Knowledge of this concept, accordingly, leads to further learning through discovery or by analogy. The final exercise in each training cycle at the Computer Station (Make Words) asks the student to type new words made of letters used in previously taught words, and the student is able to select from among the letters presented on the periphery of the screen. If an error is made, the correct letter flashes from the periphery.

Games are also included in the Writing to Read software, some of which promote speed and accuracy; others encourage increasing length of sentences. In addition, these activities add an element of fun to the program, according to its author.

Most of the creative work done by students in the program takes place at the Writing/Typing Station. Children usually begin by hunting and pecking out individual words in columns, practicing the words learned at the computer and making new words. They soon move onto typing short sentences, and eventually to writing stories. At all stages they are encouraged to edit their work, correcting errors and changing words, using the *x* key. Martin determined that children are particularly enthusiastic about using the typewriter because it renders perfect reproductions of the words they wish to write and obviates the labor of penmanship.

Martin strongly believes in the separation of writing instruction and penmanship. Although he has acknowledged that the latter skill must also be taught, he has provided little guidance on how it should be done, except to advocate the use of short, soft lead pencils. Instead, he encourages teaching children, as young as kindergarten age, to touch-type. "The speed of the typewriter," he claimed, "removes the confusion of letter formation and the delays in thought patterns because it keeps better pace with the flow of the mind" (Martin and Friedberg 1986).

Children must write in longhand, however, at the Work Journal Station where they work independently and record newly learned "cycle words." There is space for free writing in these journals as well. Throughout the program, children are encouraged to pay attention to the way words are spelled in books. With concurrent practice in phonemic writing and book reading, according to Martin, they make the transition from their invented spelling to conventional spelling.

Exposure to books takes place at the Listening Library Station, where children listen with earphones to tape recordings of stories while following the stories in books. The taped voice tells them when to turn the page so that they remain in touch with the print. This experience apparently leads children to realize that the letters they use to write their own words are the same as the letters seen in books.

Letter learning is reinforced at the Multi-Sensory Materials Station. Here children trace letters in sand trays or on emery paper, form letters with rolls of clay, and use chalk and soft lead pencils to write individual letters.

The major purpose of the Make Words Station is to teach the alphabetic principle. Children work in pairs, taking turns at showing each other pictures and having their partner spell the object in the picture with letter cards, letter stamps, magnetic letters, etc. The correct spellings are printed on the back of the picture cards, and the children act as tutors for each other.

The Writing to Read curriculum takes place daily for an hour in a learning laboratory containing each of the six work stations described above. One teacher plus an assistant is needed for each class; the assistant's main job is to guide the computer activities. Proponents of the program claim as one of its major advantages the fact that it releases teachers from spending time on phonic drills.

More recently, John Henry Martin has developed a readiness program for four-year olds to prepare them for the Writing to Read curriculum. The program, called Get Set for Writing to Read, uses the computer to teach the alphabet and basic segmentation skills. The alphabet is first introduced with the Alphabet Song, to which children listen on audio cassette while using an alphabet board to locate the letters. Next they listen to nursery rhymes and folk songs about each letter, and follow along in Verse and Rhyme Books; letters to be learned are emphasized in bold face type within the words where they appear. Children then move on to the computer, first working on the Computer Alphabet Program which introduces both uppercase and lowercase letters, along with animation and voice synthesizer, and later on the Syllable and Segment Program which illustrates the concept that many words share the same sounds and letter combinations. The program is intended to span an eighteen-week period, at the end of which time Martin maintains that children have learned a significant number of basic skills and concepts. These include: visual discrimination, letter recognition, letter names, uppercase and lowercase letters, fine motor skills, auditory memory, auditory sequencing, eye-hand coordination, keyboard familiarity, the concept that letters make words, and the concept that words contain segments or syllables that are repeated in other words. No evaluation studies have been conducted yet on Get Set.

TEACHER TRAINING

IBM provides the teacher training for Writing to Read at cost. The corporation offers three-day leadership training workshops. Teachers thus trained return to their schools and conduct two-day on-site in-service workshops for school faculty desiring training. Training consultants from IBM are also available upon request for a fee to come to schools and run follow-up workshops. Unlike some of the remedial programs, training for Writing to Read is not strictly controlled; there is no certification requirement that must be met before teaching the curriculum.

EVALUATION AND IMPLEMENTATION

The nationwide evaluation study of Writing to Read was carried out by the Educational Testing Service (ETS) (Murphy and Appel 1984). In the second year of the program (1983–1984), a core sample of 3,210 children in randomly selected schools within the participating districts was compared with a control group of 2,379 children in schools not using Writing to Read. Pre- and posttest scores on standardized reading tests were compared between the two groups for both kindergarten and first-grade students. Schools were allowed to make their own test selection from among five widely accepted nationally normed instruments. Thus reading achievement was compared across these tests, as well as between groups. Spelling achievement was measured, instead, by performance on a dictated list of ten spelling words, one for kindergarten and another for first grade, which were put together by ETS. Writing was assessed by collecting samples of writing on a single topic from three groups of children within both the experimental and control samples: kindergarten and first-grade children participating in Writing to Read in the evaluation year and first-grade students who had Writing to Read instruction while in kindergarten. Classroom teachers evaluated the writing samples, using a scoring system devised by ETS. In addition to student performance data, the evaluation included parent and teacher questionnaires.

Analyses of the data in the ETS study are complicated and the findings are difficult to interpret. In summarizing the major conclusions, however, Murphy and Appel (1984) affirm that the program functions well as a system, that children were able to handle the technology and had no difficulty adjusting to the rotational format between work stations in the learning laboratory. The evaluators also maintain that Writing to Read students in kindergarten and first grade progressed faster than comparison students in reading, that they learned to write better, and that they spelled as well as comparison students despite the lack of direct instruction in spelling. Parents, as well as teachers, apparently responded favorably to Writing to Read.

Martin (1985) acknowledges that formative evaluation studies of his program revealed that 3 to 5 percent of the children did not respond to instruction. At the same time, he contends that no incidence of dyslexia or severe reading disability was found among any of the Writing to Read students. This claim, however, may be founded less on fact than on Martin's understanding of dyslexia, which he defined as "the reversal or jumbling of letters and words in speech and writing which impairs the ability to read and to learn" (Martin and Friedberg 1986). Martin suggests that rather than dyslexia, "severe retardation in language development," as manifested by a vocabulary of less than 200 words, may have been the cause of failure in many of these children. It remains to be established, therefore, whether or not Writing to Read is effective with dyslexic children.

A recent study that relates to this question has investigated the success of Writing to Read with kindergarten children considered to be at-risk for academic failure (Markowksy 1987). The study compared the effects of combining the Writing to Read program with oral language training, aimed at increasing vocabulary knowledge, to Writing to Read instruction alone. Results of the study indicate that both at-risk and non-at-risk kindergarteners receiving oral language training made significantly greater gains in beginning reading skills, oral language skills, and writing skills, than did the comparison subjects who did not get this supplementary training. At the same time, the investigator determined that at-risk children can manage a simple word processing system and can learn letter-sound correspondences via computer with voice synthesizer.

Based on serving 120 students a day, IBM's estimated cost in 1988 for installing Writing to Read in a school, starting with an empty room, ranges from $15,000 to $18,000. The estimated cost per student over a five year period is $25.

Incentive grants given by IBM have established Writing to Read in schools throughout the country. In Tulsa, Oklahoma the program is now district-wide.

CHAPTER

Curriculum Planning for Dyslexic Students

Having discussed remedial instruction for dyslexic students in the various language arts skill areas and having presented some of the reading programs that have been developed for these students, I come now to the critical issue of determining the appropriate instructional treatment for a particular dyslexic student or group of dyslexic students. For us, as educators of dyslexic students, this issue should be one of our principal concerns, whether we are school administrators responsible for implementing and funding remedial or preventive curricula or teachers working directly with dyslexic students. It is important that all of us be involved in the decision making process and share the responsibility for the outcome of our decisions. Rather than adhering to advice from outside authorities or following trends of the publishing industry, we should know the research on specific reading disability and its treatment, and we should know our students well. Only with this combined knowledge can we begin to meet the educational requirements of these students.

Even with this knowledge, planning a language arts curriculum for a dyslexic student or students is not a simple task. A great many factors are involved, not the least being practical constraints—teacher-to-student ratio, scheduling problems, economic feasibility, and the like. This chapter discusses many of the basic considerations to keep in mind when planning instructional intervention for dyslexic students and some of the problematic issues. However, teachers, tutors, and administrators will doubtless encounter other circumstances not mentioned here while plan-ning curricula; each situation will surely have its unique challenges.

CURRICULUM COHERENCE

Several respected educators stress the need for coherence in reading and language arts curricula (Calfee 1983; Allington and Broikou 1988). Teachers should know what skills they are going to teach, why they need to teach them, how to teach them, and how these skills relate to one another.

The principle of curriculum coherence is especially relevant to the education of dyslexic students. For these students, coherence needs to oc-cur at two levels—within the remedial or special education curriculum, and between this curriculum and the regular classroom curriculum. As Richard Allington and Kathleen Broikou state, most dyslexic or at-risk children are exposed simultaneously to two different language arts curric-ula (Allington and Broikou 1988). If they are in a classroom pull-out pro-gram in school or an after-school tutoring program, they are usually re-sponsible for meeting the demands of the regular classroom curriculum. Even if enrolled in a special reading program within the school, such as one of those described in this book, they are usually exposed to a good part of what goes on in the regular classroom, or at least they should be, since the ultimate goal is for these students to succeed in the educational mainstream.

Given that dyslexic students are expected to keep up with a dual curriculum, one of our first considerations in planning remedial instruc-tion for them should be to determine the school's educational philosophy and examine its reading curriculum. Allington and Broikou point out that dyslexic students may be exposed to competing instructional philoso-phies, for instance, a meaning-based versus a code-emphasis approach. The classroom teacher may encourage using context to cue word recogni-tion, whereas the special educator or remedial teacher may discourage using context and emphasize attending to orthographic patterns in words. Viewing remedial instruction for these students within the broader con-text of the school curriculum will help us not only to develop coherence in their educational programming, but also to better understand their cur-rent academic performance patterns, inasmuch as they may have been in-fluenced by the classroom instruction provided thus far. Additionally, knowing the school's curriculum demands will help determine whether our dyslexic students may be expected eventually to function successfully within the school's mainstream. It may, in fact, become apparent that a change in school placement would be beneficial.

In order to maintain coherence across curricula for dyslexic students, there must be ongoing communication between all educational professionals involved. Remedial reading teachers or special educators must coordinate with classroom teachers, and together they must collaborate on instruction for these students, sharing their expertise, and learning about the teaching methods and activities of the other (Allington and Broikou 1988). Ideally, communication should be on a weekly basis. Specialists must become familiar with the basal series or other reading program used in the classroom, and classroom teachers must become aware of and knowledgeable about the remedial curriculum taught by specialists. Conferences may be more difficult to arrange where the specialist works with children outside the school, but in these cases they are even more important; therefore, a concerted effort must be made to find time for this purpose.

Even within a remedial curriculum, coherence needs to be monitored. Although each of the special reading programs described in this book provides a coherent curriculum structure based on a specific instructional rationale, none of them teaches all of the reading-related skills that dyslexic students need to learn. Therefore, in selecting any one of these programs, as teachers, we have to make various instructional modifications to fit our students' needs. It is important that we incorporate these additions or adaptations in a rational, cohesive manner into the larger remedial curriculum.

LEARNER CHARACTERISTICS

It goes without saying that no two dyslexic children are exactly alike in their learning patterns and achievement levels, just as nondyslexic children are not the same. In planning effective instruction for dyslexic children we must always consider their individual learning characteristics. Learner diversity may be relatively easy to handle in a one-to-one tutorial relationship; however, it is no less important, though more difficult to accommodate, when working with small groups or whole classes.

NATURE AND SEVERITY OF THE PROBLEM

Much of this information about a student will be provided by a thorough educational evaluation, and where one has been conducted, results should be available to the specialist working with the student, as well as to the student's reading or language arts teacher. Yet, even with this information, we will want to probe further to obtain a fuller sense of where the student needs help. Assessing blending and segmenting skills, for example, may not be included in the formal evaluation, and we will need to determine the student's ability in this skill when we plan a course of remedial treatment. This information can be obtained through *diagnostic teaching,* where the teacher or tutor develops informal tasks to tap the student's phonological abilities and keeps a record of the student's proficiency in the various related subskills.

Younger children entering kindergarten or first grade may not have been formally evaluated but instead may have been determined to be at-risk for dyslexia through the administration of a screening test, such as the Pre-School Screening Procedures (Slingerland 1971). School policy may designate their placement in a multisensory Slingerland class or a DISTAR class for beginning reading instruction. Those of us who teach these classes must be aware that pre-reading screening tests are not finely tuned diagnostic instruments but rather gross measures of ability; furthermore, they may have limited reliability because of the variability of developmental rates among young children (Lichenstein and Ireton 1984). Therefore, it is up to us to be sensitive to the learning differences among these students and to recognize where their needs are not being met by the curriculum.

DEVELOPMENTAL CONSIDERATIONS

Deciding which of the many published remedial programs to use with a dyslexic student or group of students is to some extent dependent upon student age and grade level, in addition to reading level. Most of these programs have been designed for a specific age range, usually children in the early elementary grades, though in some cases the range is broader; Auditory Discrimination in Depth (Lindamood and Lindamood 1975), for example, is intended for kindergarten-age through adulthood. Furthermore, some of these programs can be adapted for different ages without too much difficulty. Alphabetic Phonics, for instance, has been used effectively with adult dyslexics. Student age will be a natural consideration if we develop our own remedial curriculum; it will determine the skills we teach, and the materials and techniques we use to teach them.

Working with older dyslexic students presents particular challenges. One is providing them with sufficient experience in reading connected text, which requires finding material written at their ability level but stimulating enough in content to hold their interest. Boredom can be a problem when we attempt to engage older students in instructional routines designed for younger children. Additionally, older students may be self-conscious about performing many of the multisensory activities which we are able to use with elementary-age children, such as writing letters in the air or on sandpaper. This is more likely to be the case in a group setting; if working alone with a teacher an older student may be more willing to adopt some of these techniques. However, even in a group setting, if the teacher sets a tone of comradery and fun, she may be able to allay much of the embarrassment among older students, and if she uses her imagination, she can devise alternative activities to involve visual, auditory, and kinesthetic sensory channels.

Another important factor to consider in working with dyslexic students is the normal course of developmental change in reading behavior as a child learns to read. Fortunately we have Jeanne Chall's stage model of reading acquisition (Chall 1983b) to serve as our guide in this respect (see Chapter 1, pp. 9–12). Even though the dyslexic child's reading development has been arrested at an early stage (the decoding stage) with appropriate remedial instruction we can expect the child to progress through subsequent stages of reading acquisition in the same order, though not at the same pace, as the normally achieving child. This means that remedial reading specialists and special educators must plan instruction for dyslexic students well beyond the decoding stage, helping them to increase their sight word vocabulary and their reading fluency, encouraging them to attend to meaning as well as to print, and to use contextual as well as graphic cues to facilitate word recognition. I will say more on this subject in the section that follows.

It is also crucial that we bear in mind the changing academic demands that our dyslexic students are expected to meet as they move through the school curriculum. Reading comprehension skills become increasingly important, exposition replaces narrative as the predominant prose form, written assignments multiply, and, as the amount of reading material to be covered grows and more independent work is expected, there is a greater need for good study skills. Our job as specialists is to work together with classroom or subject area teachers in ascertaining and teaching the skills our students need.

CONCOMITANT STRENGTHS AND WEAKNESSES

Like all children, dyslexic children have various patterns of language processing abilities and personality traits, and these affect the way they perform academically. For example, in addition to phonological processing deficits, some dyslexics may have auditory perception problems that make it difficult for them to follow oral directions, visual perception problems that impair their memory for written words, poor fine-motor coordination that inhibits their handwriting development, or speech articulation difficulties that interfere with their being understood. They are very likely to have mild to severe emotional problems as a result of their dyslexia: poor self-image, defeatism, depression, sometimes denial accompanied by inappropriate bravado which tends to put off their peers. We should be sensitive to such weaknesses as we plan remedial instruction for these children.

On the other hand, many dyslexic children have remarkable abilities in areas other than written language. They may have excellent visual-spatial skills. They may be artistic. They may be imaginative and enjoy creating stories, poems, or plays. They may have a flair for dramatics. They may have a good repertoire of spoken vocabulary, despite their reading and spelling difficulties. They may be athletic. They may have a good sense of humor and a personality that wins friends. They may be extremely motivated to succeed academically and willing to work hard. We can be more effective teachers for our dyslexic students if we take advantage of their interests and their stronger abilities. We might find reading material on sports for the athlete, or plays for the drama enthusiast; or we might help the student with good visual-spatial skills to build a large sight reading vocabulary We should encourage our students to further develop abilities that may serve to motivate learning or help to compensate for their reading and spelling deficits.

EXPANDING THE CURRICULUM

No currently existing reading program meets all the instructional requirements of dyslexic students. Therefore, if we educators select any of these programs for our students, we must be prepared to add missing instructional components. Additional instruction may be called for in any of the following areas.

PHONOLOGICAL AWARENESS

Among the remedial programs for dyslexic students only Auditory Discrimination in Depth (ADD) (Lindamood and Lindamood 1975) specifically teaches phonological awareness and segmentation skills. As we know, dyslexic children, as well as adults, often lack these abilities, which are essential for proficient word decoding (see pp. 27–29). Therefore, we must ensure that training is provided in this area when it is needed.

For younger children, kindergarteners and even first-graders, this training might begin with rhyming activities and identification of initial sounds in words, along the lines of Lynette Bradley and Peter Bryant's *sound categorization tasks* (see p. 57). To further phoneme awareness and segmentation, the *Elkonin method* (see p. 55), *Williams' ABD program* (see pp. 56–57), or the *Lindamood ADD program* (see Chapter 13) can be incorporated into the curriculum. (If adopting the Elkonin method, which uses only tokens to represent letter sounds, we must provide training with letters as well.)

For older students, the Lindamood program is most appropriate for teaching the concept of phonemic segmentation. We may not choose to present the entire program but instead only some of the units, depending upon the severity of the students' phonological deficits. One of the major advantages of this program is that it provides a concrete illustration of the alphabetic principle, and substantial amounts of multisensory involvement to reinforce this principle, with a format which does not seem demeaning to older students.

WHOLE WORD RECOGNITION

Proficient reading depends on speed as well as accuracy of word identification. Most children gain automaticity in word identification through reading experience, but because they read less, dyslexic children have less opportunity to do so. Unfortunately, few of the reading programs designed for dyslexic students, or for children who might be at risk for dyslexia, provide sufficient practice in whole word recognition. Although most do treat irregularly spelled or nonphonetic high frequency words as sight words, their major focus is on developing word analysis skills. I strongly believe that provision must be made in remedial or developmental curricula to help dyslexic students build a large repertoire of words that can be instantly identified.

The most traditional approach to sight word instruction, but one which still has ample validity, is flash card drill. In this approach, the teacher (or in some cases the student) writes on index cards new words which the student has encountered or will encounter in his or her reading. The teacher asks the student to read the words aloud as each card is held up. The teacher corrects any errors, putting to one side cards with words the student missed, and continues through the pack, repeating the process until all words have been correctly read three times. The flash cards can be stored alphabetically for each student. With large groups, of course, the cards must be larger and are usually kept by the teacher. It is important that there be frequent review of these words and that none be removed from the flash card pack unless they are automatically recognized with 100 percent accuracy. Many variations of this exercise can be adopted—for example, having students take the teacher's role and quizzing each other or developing memory games with the flash cards.

The Slingerland program, as pointed out in Chapter 14 (pp. 139–145) teaches a whole word approach for text reading and uses a basal reader series for this purpose. Considerable practice is given to identifying new words in isolation before they are encountered in the text. A newer approach to increasing the speed and breadth of word recognition has been *computer assisted instruction (CAI)*. This approach is discussed at some length in Chapter 6.

READING FLUENCY

Automatic word recognition, of course, is highly relevant to fluent reading, but students also need extensive practice reading words in connected text. We should make a particular effort to see that our dyslexic students gain more experience in text reading than is provided in most remedial programs. Chapter 6 (pp. 73–77) covers several instructional approaches to increasing reading fluency, including the Slingerland approach and computer assisted instruction. However, the most effective way to increase fluent reading is to promote recreational reading. This is best accomplished by determining individual interests and finding lots of readable material to match those interests. For children with a dramatic bent, play reading can a wonderful group activity.

When the focus is on increasing fluency and speed in reading, students should be encouraged to make effective use of context. Cloze exercises are useful for this purpose. These entail replacing every fifth word or so with a blank space and asking students to read the text with as little hesitation as possible, using the context to help guess at the words that have been deleted. Naturally, the text must be well chosen and the deletions carefully considered in order to ensure reasonable guesses.

ANALOGY STRATEGIES

Although an explicit phonics approach is the preferred method for teaching dyslexic students the grapheme-phoneme correspondences, and is the method employed in most of the remedial and developmental reading programs I have described, once they can identify most letter sounds, dyslexic students should be encouraged to attend to orthographic patterns in words and begin to generalize knowledge of these patterns in identifying new words. Activities to stimulate comparison and generalization strategies can involve both real and nonsense words, for example: If *bait* says "bait," what does *trait* say? What does *chait* say? These exercises can be conducted with manipulable letters, as in the Lindamood program (see p. 134), as well as in writing.

READING COMPREHENSION SKILLS

As I emphasized in Chapter 7, any effective reading curriculum must include reading comprehension instruction; this is particularly so for dyslexic students. Once these students have learned the basic grapheme-phoneme correspondences and reached a reasonable degree of decoding proficiency, it is important to help them "unglue from print," as Jeanne Chall (1983b) has expressed it. At this juncture, we need to encourage them to pay increasing attention to meaning as they read, to involve both top-down and bottom-up strategies and apply a more interactive approach to processing text.

Many of the newer perspectives on reading comprehension and instructional approaches to enhance comprehension are discussed in Chapter 7: effective application of background knowledge, employment of metacognitive strategies, and guided learning, to name a few. Among the remedial and developmental reading programs described in this book, only three give any appreciable consideration to teaching comprehension skills—Enfield and Greene's Project Read, Calfee's Project READ, and Corrective Reading (DISTAR)—and even these programs could benefit from a broader approach to comprehension instruction. Readers should refer to Chapter 7 for suggestions on instructional strategies for promoting text comprehension which they might wish to incorporate in reading curricula for their dyslexic students.

Two additional suggestions are offered in regard to teaching comprehension skills. The first is that comprehension instruction should be introduced into the curriculum as early as conceivably possible, in terms of both age and reading level. The second is that children should have early experience with expository text in order to prepare them for the content area material they will begin to encounter in fourth grade.

VOCABULARY DEVELOPMENT

None of the remedial programs deriving from the Orton-Gillingham approach devote much attention to increasing knowledge of word meanings, with the exception of Enfield and Greene's Project Read which teaches word roots and affixes to fourth- through ninth-grade students. At the highest level of its decoding strand, Corrective Reading, the extension of the DISTAR direct instruction model, teaches 600 vocabulary words by defining them and presenting them in text; however, there is no theoretical rationale behind the selection of these particular words (see p. 173). Among all the reading programs described in this book, only Calfee's Project READ presents a conceptual framework for vocabulary development. This program places major emphasis on forming semantic relationships between words (see pp. 181–182), but also includes instruction in morphology or meaningful word parts.

Because they read less, dyslexic students have even greater need for vocabulary instruction than normally achieving students. Surprisingly, there is no consensus on the best way to teach vocabulary to either good readers or disabled readers. At the same time, there is no indication from research that dyslexic students require a different approach to vocabulary instruction than nondyslexic students.

After several years of conducting research on vocabulary development, Margaret McKeown and Isabel Beck proposed an instructional program incorporating many of the principles and components they found to be most effective for increasing knowledge of word meanings (McKeown and Beck 1988). These investigators made several determinations about effective vocabulary instruction. One is that new words to be learned need to be presented in a variety of contexts and taught through a variety of activities, such as associating words with synonyms or definitions, relating words with different contexts, generating new contexts for words, and comparing and contrasting words on various semantic dimensions. Another determination is that new words require frequent and numerous encounters (at least ten) to be learned well. Additionally, they maintain that not all unfamiliar words that students encounter deserve to be learned in this "rich" way, but some only well enough to make sense of the text in which they appear. Although they believe that the selection of words to be taught should be based on the classroom curriculum and consider basal readers to be major sources of new words, McKeown and Beck criticize basal reading programs for their "egalitarian treatment of all categories of words." They suggest that teachers look for unfamiliar words in forthcoming lessons and decide which among them would be useful to their students, thereby warranting a "rich" instructional approach. Other unknown words would be taught in a "narrow" way. Lastly, McKeown and Beck believe that to gain greater facility with new vocabulary words, students need to be encouraged to use these words beyond the classroom. To motivate extended use of new vocabulary, McKeown and Beck devised a game called Word Wizard in which students earn points by reporting on contexts where they have encountered words that they have studied or by using these words in their own speech or writing.

The major features of McKeown and Beck's proposed vocabulary development program would seem to be easily implemented with dyslexic students. If a basal series is not being used, new words can be culled from trade books or other support materials provided by teachers who would scan the materials ahead of time for unfamiliar words and teach the words that they chose. For nonreaders, teachers can select words for instruction from stories or exposition read aloud to students.

WRITTEN EXPRESSION

Chapter 10 discusses composition instruction for dyslexic students, which I have indicated is all but neglected in the reading programs that have been designed for these students. I therefore refer readers to this chapter for suggestions on instructional components that may need to be incorporated in curriculum planning for their dyslexic students. Despite, or perhaps because of, the very systematic, skills oriented instruction provided in these reading programs, we need to foster self-expression and creativity in dyslexic students' writing.

The main point I wish to stress here is that dyslexic children and adolescents should be encouraged to write, regardless of spelling problems or any other mechanical difficulties they experience. Furthermore, writing should be encouraged from the moment these students begin remedial or preventive instruction, even if it entails only one or two words. This writing experience should be individualized. No effort should be made by the teacher to correct errors, although she should be available to help students seeking assistance. Students should not be asked to share their written products, unless they seem eager to do so. Although group writing, teacher modeling, dictated composition, and other writing experiences have a place in their remedial or developmental language arts curricula, personal writing experiences help dyslexic students develop a sense of ownership or control over their writing. Therefore, a short period should be allotted several times a week for individual writing. The teacher may offer a story-starting theme, but should not insist that it be followed; indeed, the teacher should urge students to initiate their own themes. Students can be given folders in which to keep this written work; the folders might receive very personal titles. Motivated students who wish to share their personal writing can be encouraged to bind their work into a book form and perhaps illustrate their stories or poems.

PRACTICAL CONSIDERATIONS

One of the first factors to consider in planning a reading curriculum for dyslexic students is the *academic setting* in which they will be receiving remedial treatment; this may be a reading clinic or private office outside school, a reading specialist's office within school, a resource room, a special self-contained classroom, or a regular classroom. A second basic consideration is the *number of students* for which you are planning remedial instruction; this may range from one to any number. Closely related to this factor is the teacher-to-student ratio in the remedial curriculum, whether the teacher or clinician will be working with one student at a time, with small groups of students, or with whole classes. *Scheduling time* for pupils within school or after school may also be a determining factor.

Another very important consideration in curriculum planning for dyslexic students is the *school's reading program,* whether it uses a basal reader program and how closely it adheres to this program. *Attitudinal factors* also play an important role in implementing remedial instruction: the school administration's level of concern for disabled readers; teachers' views on reading instruction and reading underachievement; and parents' feelings about their children's reading problems and what to do about them.

Teacher training is a pivotal element in remedial education. Training requirements vary greatly across remedial programs in terms of rigor, time, and cost. This information is provided in the section entitled "Teacher Training" in each of the chapters describing these programs.

In addition to teacher training, which can be one of the largest expenses in program implementation, equipment and materials' costs must be weighed; here too, there is tremendous variation among reading programs. Writing to Read, for example, which I consider to be a developmental or preventive program rather than a remedial program, is by far the most expensive to implement because of the technical equipment required (computers, typewriters, work stations, etc.), as well as student materials. Recipe for Reading, in marked contrast, requires purchasing only a teacher's manual. However, we must be aware that this program and most of the other Orton-Gillingham derivative programs require that teachers make many of the instructional materials themselves, which can be costly in terms of time. Although implementation costs are cited for some programs in the section entitled "Program Evaluation and Implementation" at the end of each of the program chapters, I advise readers to contact publishers and teacher training centers directly to gain further information and up-to-date figures on the expenses involved.

TEACHERS AS RESEARCHERS

A final point I would like to make is that those of us who work with dyslexic children and adolescents should take a greater leadership role than we have in the past in planning their language arts curriculum. This requires that we know the research on dyslexia and its treatment and that we keep abreast of recent developments in teaching methods for treating dyslexia, including the application of computer technology. Having this knowledge will enable us to influence educational change rather than leaving curriculum decision-making to administrators not as closely involved with these students as we are. Gaining this knowledge, of course, demands a substantial expenditure of time and effort, even more than we already give to our field; it entails attending conferences, taking courses after work, over weekends, or during summers, and keeping up with research journals and new publications.

Besides using the research findings of others to judge the potential value of instructional approaches and programs for our dyslexic students, we ourselves need to become researchers. We can begin by documenting and evaluating our own applications of these teaching methods and disseminating this information, thereby adding to the research base. We may develop new teaching methods and techniques in our ongoing work with dyslexic students; these too should be evaluated for their effectiveness, preferably with well controlled studies (note the unfortunate absence of controls in so much of the research cited in this book) and the results shared with our colleagues. The results, when successful, should also be available to administrators responsible for funding and implementing new programs. The history of Project Read (Enfield and Greene) in Minnesota (see Chapter 16) is an excellent example of how teachers can initiate and bring about effective curriculum change to prevent reading failure.

References

Aaron, P. G., and Phillips, S. 1986. A decade of research with dyslexic college students. *Annals of Dyslexia* 36:44–68.

Abernathy, E. W., Martin, R. C., and Caramazza, A. 1982. The role of phonological working memory in written sentence comprehension. Paper presented at the annual meeting of the Eastern Psychological Association.

Aho, M. S. 1967. Teaching spelling to children with specific language disability. *Academic Therapy* 3:45–50.

Allington, R. L., and Broikou, K. A. 1988. Development of shared knowledge: A new role for classroom and special teachers. *The Reading Teacher* 41:806–11.

Anderson, R. C. 1977. The notion of schema and the educational enterprise: General discussion of the conference. In *Schooling and the Acquisition of Knowledge,* ed. R. C. Anderson, R. J. Spiro, and W. E. Montaque, 50–79. Hillsdale, NJ: Lawrence Erlbaum Associates.

Anderson, R. C., Hiebert, E. H., Scott, J. A., and Wilkinson, I. A. G. 1984. *Becoming a Nation of Readers.* Washington, D.C.: National Institute of Education.

Arkes, J. 1986. The ABCs of Project Read. Bloomington, MN: Bloomington Public Schools.

Askov, E., and Greff, N. 1975. Handwriting: Copying versus tracing as the most effective type of practice. *Journal of Educational Research* 69:96–98.

Au, K. H.-P., Tharp, R. G., Crowell, D. C., Jordan, C., Speidel, G. E., and Calkins, R. 1985. The role of research in a successful reading program. In *Reading Education: Foundations for a Literate America,* ed. J. Osborn, P. T. Wilson, and R. C. Anderson, 275–292. Lexington, MA: D. C. Heath.

Backman, J., Bruck, M., Hebert, M., and Seidenberg, M. S. 1984. Acquisition and use of spelling-sound correspondences in reading. *Journal of Experimental Child Psychology* 38:114–133.

Bain, A. M. 1986. Written language: Test results and informal assessment data. Paper presented at the Thirteenth Annual Conference of the New York Branch of The Orton Dyslexia Society, March, 1986.

Baker, L., and Brown, A. L. 1984. Metacognitive skills in reading. In *Handbook of Reading Research,* ed. P. D. Pearson, 353–94. New York: Longman.

Ball, E. W., and Blachman, B. A. 1987. A reading readiness program with an emphasis on phoneme segmentation. Paper presented at the 38th Annual Conference of The Orton Dyslexia Society, November, 1987.

Ballesteros, D. A., and Royal, N. L. 1981. Slingerland-SLD instruction as a winning voluntary magnet program. *Bulletin of The Orton Society* 31:199–211.

Bandura, A. 1982. Self-efficiency mechanism in human agency. *American Psychologist* 37(2):122–47.

Bannatyne, A. 1971. *Language, Reading, and Learning Disabilities.* Springfield, Il.: Charles C Thomas.

Barenbaum, E. M. 1983. Writing in the special class. *Topics in Learning and Learning Disabilities* 3:12–20.

Barger, E. J. 1982. The effect of the Glass Analysis technique for decoding words on the reading and spelling achievement of 7 to 10-year-old remedial readers. Ph.D. diss., George Washington University, Washington, D. C.

Barron, R. W. 1980. Visual and phonological strategies in reading and spelling. In *Cognitive Processes in Spelling,* ed. U. Frith, 195–213. New York: Academic Press.

Bartlett, E. J. 1979. Curriculum, concepts of literacy, and social class. In *Theory and Practice of Early Reading, Vol. 2,* ed. L. B. Resnick and P. A. Weaver, 227-42. Hillsdale, NJ: Lawrence Erlbaum Associates.

Bateman, B. 1979. Teaching reading to learning disabled and other hard-to-teach children. In *Theory and Practice of Early Reading: Vol. 1,* ed. L. B. Resnick and P. A. Weaver, 227–59. Hillsdale, NJ: Lawrence Erlbaum Associates.

Beck, I. L., and McCaslin, E. S. 1978. An analysis of dimensions that affect the development of code-breaking ability in eight beginning reading programs. Pittsburgh, PA: Learning Research and Development Center, University of Pittsburgh. (ERIC Document Reproduction Service No. ED 155 585).

Beck, I. L., Omanson, R. C., and McKeown, M. G. 1982. An instructional redesign of reading lessons: Effects on comprehension. *Reading Research Quarterly* 17:462–81.

Becker, W. C. 1977. Teaching reading and language to the disadvantaged—What we have learned from field research. *Harvard Educational Review* 47:518–43.

Bell, N. 1986. *Visualizing and Verbalizing for Language Comprehension and Thinking.* Paso Robles, CA: Academy of Reading Publications.

Benton, A. L. 1985. Visual factors in dyslexia: An unresolved issue. In *Understanding Learning Disabilities: International and Multidisciplinary Views,* ed. D. Duane and C. K. Leong, 87–96. New York: Oxford University Press.

Berlin, D. 1887. *Eine Besondere Art der Wrotblindheit (Dyslexie).* Wiesbaden: J. F. Bergmann.

Berliner, D. 1981. Academic learning time and reading achievement. In *Comprehension and Teaching,* ed. J. T. Guthrie, 203–26. Newark, DE: International Reading Association.

Berman, P., and McLaughlin, M. 1975. Federal programs supporting educational change, Vol. 4: The findings in review (Report No. R-1589/4). Santa Monica, CA: Rand Corp. (ERIC Document Reproduction Service No. ED 108 330.)

Biemiller, A. 1970. The development of the use of graphic and contextual information as children learn to read. *Reading Research Quarterly* 6:75–96.

Birch, H. G. 1962. Dyslexia and maturation of visual function. *Reading Disability: Progress and Research Needs in Dyslexia,* ed. J. Money, 161–70. Baltimore, MD: The Johns Hopkins University Press.

Birch, H. G., and Belmont, L. 1964. Auditory-visual integration in normal and retarded readers. *American Journal of Orthopsychiatry* 34:852–861.

Birsh, J. 1988. Multisensory teaching and discovery learning in Alphabetic Phonics. Paper presented at the Fifteenth Annual Conference of the New York Branch of The Orton Dyslexia Society, March 5, 1988.

Bissex, G. L. 1980. *Genius at Work: A Child Begins to Write and Read.* Cambridge, MA: Harvard University Press.

Blachman, B. A. 1983. Are we assessing the linguistic factors critical in early reading? *Annals of Dyslexia* 33:91–109.

Blachman, B. A. 1984. Language analysis skills and early reading acquisition. In *Language Learning Disabilities in School-Age Children,* ed. G. P. Wallach and K. G. Butler, 271–87. Baltimore, MD: Williams and Wilkins.

Blank, M. 1985. A word is a word—or is it? In *Biobehavioral Measures of Dyslexia,* ed. D. B. Gray and J. F. Kavanagh, 261–78. Parkton, MD: York Press.

Blann, M. In press. *The Sounds of Sentences.* Winooski, VT: Laureate Learning.

Blank, M., and P. Bruskin. 1982. Sentences and non-content words: Missing ingredients in reading instruction. *Annals of Dyslexia* 32:103–21.

Bloomfield, L., Barnhart, C. L., and Barnhart, R. K. 1965. *Let's Read.* Cambridge, MA: Educators Publishing Service.

BOCES Regional Office of Planning and Evaluation. 1980. A study of the South Huntington School District Slingerland Program. Suffolk County, NY: Author.

Boder, E. 1971. Developmental dyslexia: A diagnostic screening procedure based on three characteristic patterns of reading and spelling. In *Learning Disorders: Vol. 4,* ed. B. D. Bateman, 298–342. Seattle, WA: Special Child Publications.

Boder, E., and Jarrico, S. 1982. *The Boder Test of Reading-Spelling Patterns.* New York. Grune and Stratton.

Boettcher, J. V. 1983. Computer-based education: Classroom application and benefits for the learning disabled. *Annals of Dyslexia* 33:203–19.

Bradley, L. 1985. Dissociation of reading and spelling behavior. In *Understanding Learning Disabilities: International and Multidisciplinary Views,* ed. D. Duane and C. K. Leong, 65–85. New York: Plenum Press.

Bradley, L., and Bryant, P. E. 1979. Independence of reading and spelling in backward and normal readers. *Developmental Medical Child Neurology* 21:504–14.

Bradley, L., and Bryant, P. E. 1983. Categorizing sounds and learning to read: A causal connection. *Nature* 301:419–21.

Bradley, L., and Bryant, P. E. 1985. *Rhyme and Reason in Reading and Spelling.* Ann Arbor, MI: University of Michigan Press.

Brady, S., and Fowler, A. E. 1988. Phonological precursors to reading acquisition. In *Preschool Prevention of Reading Failure,* ed. R. L. Masland and M. W. Masland, 204–215. Parkton, MD: York Press.

Brady, S., Shankweiler, D., and Mann, V. 1983. Speech perception and memory coding in relation to reading ability. *Journal of Experimental Child Psychology* 35:345–67.

Brendt, R. S. 1983. Phonological coding and written sentence comprehension. *Annals of Dyslexia* 33:55–66.

Brightman, M. F. 1986. *An Evaluation of the Impact of the Alphabetic Phonics Program in the Kinkaid School from 1983–1985.* Houston, TX: Neuhaus Foundation.

Brown, A. L., Palinscar, A. S., and Armbruster, B. B. 1984. Instructing comprehension-fostering activities in interactive learning situations. In *Learning and Comprehension of Text,* ed. M. Mandl, N. L. Stein, and T. Trebasso, 255–86. Hillsdale, NJ: Lawrence Erlbaum Associates.

Bruck, M. 1988. The word recognition and spelling of dyslexic children. *Reading Research Quarterly* 23:52–68.

Bryant, N. D. 1965. Some principles of remedial instruction for dyslexia. *The Reading Teacher* 18:567–72.

Bryant, N. D. 1985. Dyslexia. In *International Encyclopedia of Education,* ed. T. Husen and I. N. Postlethwaite, 1470–75. Oxford: Pergoman Press.

Bryant, N. D. and others. 1980. The effects of some instructional variables on the learning of handicapped and nonhandicapped populations: A review. *Integrative Reviews of Research: Vol. I,* 1–70. New York: Teachers College, Institute for the Study of Learning Disabilities.

Bryant, P. E. 1968. Comments on the design of developmental studies of cross-modal matching and cross-modal transfer. *Cortex* 4:127–8.

Bryant, S. 1979. Relative effectiveness of visual-auditory versus visual-auditory-kinesthetic-tactile procedures for teaching sight words and letter sounds to young disabled readers. Ed.D. diss., Teachers College, New York.

Byrne, B. 1981. Deficient syntactic control in poor readers: Is a weak phonetic memory code responsible? *Applied Psycholinguistics* 2:201–12.

Calfee, R. 1976. Letter addressed to Mr. and Mrs. Charles Lindamood.

Calfee, R. 1983. The mind of the dyslexic. *Annals of Dyslexia* 33:9–28.

Calfee, R. and Associates. 1981–1984. *The Book: Components of Reading Instruction.* Unpublished manuscript.

Calfee, R., and Henry, M. K., 1985. Project READ: An inservice model for training classroom teachers in effective reading instruction. In *The Effective Teaching of Reading: Theory and Practice,* ed. J. Hoffman, 143–60. Newark, DE: International Reading Association.

Calfee, R., Henry, M., and Funderberg, J. 1988. A model for school change. In *Changing School Reading Programs,* ed. J. Samuels and D. Pearson, 121–41. Newark, DE: International Reading Association.

Calfee, R., Lindamood, P., and Lindamood, C. 1973. Acoustic-phonetic skills and reading; Kindergarten through twelfth grade. *Journal of Educational Psychology* 64:293–98.

Calfee, R., and Piontkowski, D. C. 1981. The reading diary: Acquisition of decoding. *Reading Research Quarterly* 3:346–73.

Canney, G., and Winograd, P. 1979. Schemata for reading and reading comprehension performance (Technical Report No. 120) Center for the Study of Reading. (ERIC Document Reproduction Service No. ED 169 520.

Carpenter, D. 1983. Spelling error profiles of able and disabled readers. *Journal of Learning Disabilities* 16, 102–4.

Carroll, J. B. 1963. A model of school learning. *Teachers College Record* 64:723–33.

Chall, J. S. 1978. A decade of research on reading and learning disabilities. In *What Research Has to Say about Reading.* ed. J. Samuels, 22–31. Newark, DE: International Reading Association.

Chall, J. S. 1983a. *Learning to Read: The Great Debate.* New York: McGraw-Hill.

Chall, J. S. 1983b. *Stages of Reading Development:* New York: McGraw-Hill.

Childs, S. B., and Childs, R. S. 1971. *Sound Spelling.* Cambridge, MA: Educators Publishing Service.

Childs, S. B., and Childs, R. S. 1973. *The Childs Spelling System: The Rules.* Cambridge, MA: Educators Publishing Service.

Chomsky, C. 1979. Approaching reading through invented spelling. In *Theory and Practice of Early Reading,* ed. L. B. Resnick and P. A. Weaver, 43–65. Hillsdale, NJ: Lawrence Erlbaum Associates.

Cicci, R. 1983. Disorders of written language. In *Progress in Learning Disabilities: Vol. 5,* ed. H. Myklebust, 207–32. New York: Grune and Stratton.

Clark, F. L., Deshler, D. D., Schumaker, J. B., Aley, G. R., and Warner, M. M. 1984. Visual imagery and self-questioning: Strategies to improve comprehension of written material. *Journal of Learning Disabilities* 17:145–49.

Cone, T. E., Wilson, L. R., Bradley, C. M., and Reese, J. H. 1985. Characteristics of LD students in Iowa: An empirical investigation. *Learning Disability Quarterly* 3(3):211–20.

Connors, C. K. 1978. Critical review of "Electroencephalographic and neuropsychological studies in dyslexia." In *Dyslexia: An Appraisal of Current Knowledge,* ed. A. L. Benton and D. Pearl, 253–61. New York: Oxford University Press.

Cooper, C., and O'Dell, L. 1977. *Evaluating Writing.* Urbana, IL: National Council of Teachers of English.

Cox, A. R. 1977. *Situation Spelling.* Cambridge, MA: Educators Publishing Service.

Cox, A. R. 1983. Programming for teachers of dyslexics. *Annals of Dyslexia* 33:221–233.

Cox, A. R. 1984. *Structures and Techniques.* Cambridge, MA: Educators Publishing Service.

Cox, A. R. 1985. Alphabetic Phonics: An organization and expansion of Orton-Gillingham. *Annals of Dyslexia* 35:187–98.

Cronbach, L. J., and Snow, R. B. 1976. *Aptitude and Instructional Methods.* New York: Irvington.

DeCecco, J. P. 1968. *The Psychology of Learning and Instruction.* Englewood Cliffs, NJ: Prentice-Hall.

Denckla, M. B. 1977. Minimal brain dysfunction and dyslexia: Beyond diagnosis by exclusion. In *Topics in Child Neurology.* ed. M. E. Blau, I. Rapin, and M. Kinsbourne, 112–125. New York: Spectrum Publishers.

Denckla, M. B. 1978. Critical review of "Electroencephalographic and neuropsychological studies in dyslexia." In *Dyslexia: An Appraisal of Current Knowledge,* ed. A. L. Benton and D. Pearl, 243–44. New York: Oxford University Press.

Denckla, M. B. 1986. Issues of overlap and heterogeneity in dyslexia. In *Biobehavioral Measures of Dyslexia,* ed. D. B. Gray and J. F. Kavanagh, 41–46. Parkton, MD: York Press.

Denckla, M. B. 1987. Applications of disconnection concepts to developmental dyslexia. *Annals of Dyslexia* 27:51–63.

Denckla, M. B., LeMay, M., and Chapman, C. A. 1985. Few CT scan abnormalities found even in neurologically impaired learning disabled children. *Journal of Learning Disabilities* 18:132–6.

Denckla, M. B., and Rudel, R. G. 1976a. Naming of object-drawings by dyslexic and other learning disabled children. *Brain and Language* 3:1–15.

Denckla, M. B., and Rudel, R. G. 1976b. Rapid automatized naming (R.A.N.): Dyslexia differentiated from other learning disabilities. *Neuropsychologia* 14:471–79.

Dobson, L. 1985. Learn to read by writing: A practical program for reluctant readers. *Teaching Exceptional Children* 18:30–36.

Doehring, D. G. 1984. Subtyping of reading disorders: Implications for remediation. *Annals of Dyslexia* 34:205–16.

Dolch, E. W. 1952. *Basic Sight Vocabulary Cards.* Champaign, IL: Garrard Publishing Co.

Duane, D. D. 1983a. Underachievement in written language: Auditory aspects. In *Progress in Learning Disabilities: Vol. 5,* ed. H. H. Myklebust, 177–206. New York: Grune and Stratton.

Duane, D. D. 1983b. Neurobiological correlates of reading disorders. *Journal of Educational Research* 77:5–15.

Duffy, F. H., Denckla, M. B., Bartels, R. H. and Sandini, G. 1980. Dyslexia: Regional differences in brain electrical activity by topographic mapping. *Annals of Neurology* 7:412–20.

Durkin, D. 1978–1979. What classroom observations reveal about reading comprehension instruction. *Reading Research Quarterly* 14:481–533.

Durkin, D. 1984. Do basal readers teach reading comprehension? In *Learning to Read in American Schools,* ed. R. C. Anderson, J. Osborn, and R. J. Tierney, 63–114. New York: Academic Press.

Eckwall, E. E., and Shanker, J. L. 1983. *Diagnosis and Remediation of the Disabled Reader.* Boston: Allyn and Bacon.

Ehri, L. 1979. Linguistic insight: Threshold of reading acquisition. In *Reading Research: Advances in Theory and Practice: Vol. 2,* ed. G. E. MacKinnon and T. G. Waller, 63–114. New York: Academic Press.

Ehri, L. 1985. Learning to read and spell. Paper presented at the Annual Meeting of the American Educational Research Association, March, 1985, Chicago.

Elkonin, D. B. 1963. The psychology of mastering the elements of reading. In *Educational Psychology in the U.S.S.R.,* ed. B. Simon and J. Simon, 165–79. London: Routledge and Kegan Paul.

Elkonin, D. B. 1973. U.S.S.R. In *Comparative Reading,* ed. J. Downing, 551–79. New York: MacMillan.

Enfield, M. L. 1976. An alternate classroom approach to meeting special learning needs of children with reading problems. Ph.D. diss., University of Minnesota, Minneapolis, MN.

Enfield, M. L., and Greene, V. E. 1981. There is a skeleton in every closet. *Bulletin of The Orton Society* 31:189–98.

Enfield, M. L., and Greene, V. E. 1983. An evaluation of the results of standardized testing of elementary Project Read and SLD students based on district wide tests administered in October, 1983. Bloomington, MN: Bloomington Public Schools.

Enfield, M. L., and Greene, V. E. 1985. *Project Read Practical Spelling Guide.* Bloomington, MN: Bloomington Public Schools.

Engelmann, S., Becker, W. C., Hanner, S., and Johnson, G. 1978. *Corrective Reading: Decoding B.* Chicago: Science Research Associates.

Engelmann, S., Becker, W. C., Hanner, S., and Johnson, G. 1980. *Corrective Reading Series Guide.* Chicago: Science Research Associates.

Engelmann, S., and Bruner, E. C. 1983. *Reading Mastery I and II: DISTAR Reading.* Chicago: Science Research Associates.

Epstein, M. H., and Cullinan, D. 1981. Project EXCEL: A behaviorally-oriented educational program for learning disabled pupils. *Education and Treatment of Children* 4:357–73.

Farnham-Diggory, S. 1986a. Commentary: Time, now, for a little serious complexity. In *Handbook of Cognitive, Social, and Neurological Aspects of Learning Disabilities: Vol 1,* ed. S. P. Cecci, 123–60. Hillsdale, NJ: Lawrence Erlbaum Associates.

Farnham-Diggery, S. 1986b. Introduction to the third revised edition. In *The Writing Road to Reading,* by R. B. Spalding and W. T. Spalding, 9–20. New York: Quill/William Morrow.

Fernald, G. M. 1943. *Remedial Techniques in Basic School Subjects*. New York: McGraw-Hill.

Fernald, G. M., and Keller, H. 1921. The effect of kinesthetic factors in development of word recognition in the case of non-readers. *Journal of Educational Research* 4:355–77.

Feuerstein, R. 1979. *The Dynamic Assessment of Retarded Performers: The Learning-Potential Assessment Device, Theory, Instruments, and Techniques*. Baltimore: University Park Press.

Fleisher, L. S., Jenkins, J. R., and Pany, D. 1979. Effects on poor readers' comprehension of training in rapid decoding. *Reading Research Quarterly* 15:30–48.

Forrell, E. R., and Hood, J. 1985. A longitudinal study of two groups of children with early reading problems. *Annals of Dyslexia* 35:97–116.

Fox, B., and Routh, D. K. 1980. Phonemic analysis and severe reading disability in children. *Journal of Psycholinguistic Research* 9:115–19.

Fox, B., and Routh, D. K. 1983. Reading disability, phonemic analysis and dysphonetic spelling: A follow-up study. *Journal of Clinical Child Psychology* 12:28–32.

Fox, B., and Routh, D. K. 1984. Phonemic analysis and synthesis as word attack skills: Revisited. *Journal of Educational Psychology* 76:1059–64.

Frankiewicz, R. G. 1984. An evaluation of the impact of the Alphabetic Phonics Program in Cypress Fairbanks Independent School District from 1981 through 1984. Houston, TX: Neuhaus Foundation.

Frankiewicz, R. G. 1985. An evaluation of the Alphabetic Phonics Program offered in the one-to-one mode. Houston, TX: Neuhaus Education Center.

Frauenheim, J. G., and Heckerl, J. R. 1983. A longitudinal study of psychological and achievement test performance in severe dyslexic adults. *Journal of Learning Disabilities* 16:339–47.

Frederiksen, J. R., and others. 1983. A componential approach to training reading skills. Final report. Cambridge, MA: Bolt, Beranek, and Newman.

Fries, C. C., Wilson, R. G., and Rudolph, M. K. 1966. *Merrill Linguistic Readers*. Columbus, OH: Charles E. Merrill.

Frith, U. 1986. Beneath the surface of developmental dyslexia. In *Surface Dyslexia*, ed. K. E. Patterson, J. C. Marshall, and M. Coltheart, 301–30. Hillsdale, NJ: Lawrence Erlbaum Associates.

Frith, U., and Frith, C. 1983. Relationships between reading and spelling. In *Orthography, Reading, and Dyslexia*, ed. J. P. Kavanagh and R. L. Venezky, 287–95. Baltimore: University Park Press.

Furner, B. A. 1983. Developing handwriting ability: A perceptual learning process. *Topics in Learning and Learning Disabilities* 3:41–54.

Galaburda, A. M. 1983. Developmental dyslexia: Current anatomical research. *Annals of Dyslexia* 33:41–54.

Galaburda, A. M. 1985. Developmental dyslexia: A review of biological interactions. *Annals of Dyslexia* 35:21–34.

Galaburda, A. M., and Kemper, T. L. 1979. Cytoarchitectonic abnormalities in developmental dyslexia: A case study. *Annals of Neurology* 6:94–100.

Gambrell, L. B., and Bales, R. J. 1986. Mental imagery and the comprehension-monitoring performance of fourth- and fifth-grade poor readers. *Reading Research Quarterly* 21:454–64.

Ganschow, L. 1984. Analysis of written language of a language learning disabled (dyslexic) college student and instructional implications. *Annals of Dyslexia* 34:271–84.

Gates, A. I. 1927. *The Improvement of Reading: A Program of Diagnostic and Remedial Methods*. New York: MacMillan.

Gerber, M., and Hall, R. J. 1987. Information processing approaches to studying spelling deficiencies. *Journal of Learning Disabilities* 20:34–42.

German, D. 1984. Diagnosis of word-finding disorders in children with learning disabilities. *Journal of Learning Disabilities* 17:353–59.

Gersten, R., Woodward, J., and Darch, C. 1986. Direct Instruction: A research-based approach to curriculum design and teaching. *Exceptional Children* 53:17–31.

Geschwind, N. 1986. The biology of dyslexia: The unfinished manuscript. In *Biobehavioral Measures of Dyslexia*, ed. D. B. Gray and J. F. Kavanagh, 21–24. Parkton, MD: York Press.

Geschwind, N., and Behan, P. 1982. Left-handedness: Association with immune disease, migraine, and developmental learning disorder. *Proceedings of the National Academy of Science* 79:5097–5100.

Gillingham, A., and Stillman, B. 1960. *Remedial Training for Children with Specific Disability in Reading, Writing, and Penmanship*. Cambridge, MA: Educators Publishing Service.

Gittelman, R. 1983. Treatment of reading disorders. In *Developmental Neuropsychiatry*, ed. M. Rutter, 520–41. New York: Guilford Press.

Glass, G. G., and Glass, E. W. 1976. *Glass Analysis for Decoding Only: Teachers Guide*. Garden City, NY: Easier to Learn.

Glass, G. G., and Glass, E. W. 1978a. *Glass Analysis for Decoding Only: Easy Starts Kit*. Garden City, NY: Easier to Learn.

Glass, G. G., and Glass, E. W. 1978b. *Glass Analysis for Decoding Only: Quick and Easy Alphabet Program*. Garden City, NY: Easier to Learn.

Godfrey, J. J., Syrdal-Lasky, A. K., Millaj, K. K., and Knox, C. M. 1981. Performance of dyslexic children on speech perception tests. *Journal of Experimental Child Psychology* 32:401–24.

Goodman, K. 1967. Reading: A psycholinguistic guessing game. *Journal of the Reading Specialist* 6:126–35.

Gough, P. B., and Tunmer, W. E. 1986. Decoding, reading, and reading disability. *Remedial and Special Education* 7:6–10.

Grant, S. M. 1985. The kinesthetic approach to teaching: Building a foundation. *Journal of Learning Disabilities* 18:455–62.

Graves, D. 1978. *Balance the Basics: Let Them Write*. New York: Ford Foundation.

Graves, D. 1983. *Writing: Teachers and Children at Work*. Exeter, NH: Heinemann.

Graves, D. 1985. All children can write. *Learning Disability Focus* 1:36–43.

Greene, V. E., and M. L. Enfield. 1981. *Project Read Affix Guide*. Bloomington, MN: Bloomington Public Schools.

Greene, V. E., and Enfield, M. L. 1983. *There's a Skeleton in Every Closet*. Bloomington, MN: Bloomington Public Schools.

Greene, V. E., and Enfield, M. L. 1985a. *Project Read Reading Guide: Phase I*. Bloomington, MN: Bloomington Public Schools.

Greene, V. E., and Enfield, M. L. 1985b. *Project Read Reading Guide: Phase II*. Bloomington, MN: Bloomington Public Schools.

Guthrie, J. T. 1978. Principles of instruction: A critique of Johnson's "Remedial approaches to dyslexia." In *Dyslexia: An Appraisal of Current Knowledge*, ed. A. L. Benton and D. Pearl, 425–35. New York: Oxford University Press.

Haines, L. P., and Leong, C. K. 1983. Coding processes in skilled and less skilled readers. *Annals of Dyslexia* 33:67–89.

Hammill, D. D., and Larsen, S. C. 1978. *The Test of Written Language*. Austin, TX: Pro-Ed.

Hanna, P. R., Hodges, R. E., Hanna, J. L., and Rudolph, E. H. 1966. *Phoneme-Grapheme Correspondence as Cues to Spelling Improvement*. Washington, D. C.: Department of Health, Education, and Welfare, Office of Education.

Hansen, J. 1981. The effects of inference training and practice on young children's reading comprehension. *Reading Research Quarterly* 16:391–417.

Hansen, J., and Pearson, P. D. 1983. An instructional study: Improving the inferential comprehension of good and poor fourth-grade readers. *Journal of Educational Psychology* 75:821–29.

Harber, J. R. 1983. The effects of illustrations on the reading performance of learning disabled and normal children. *Learning Disability Quarterly* 6:55–60.

Hardyck, C., and Petrinovich, L. F. 1977. Left-handedness. *Psychological Bulletin* 84:385–404.

Haring, N. G., and Bateman, B. 1977. *Teaching the Learning Disabled Child*. Englewood Cliffs, NJ: Prentice-Hall.

Haring, N. G., Bateman, B., and Carnine, D. 1977. Direct Instruction—DISTAR. In *Teaching the Learning Disabled Child*, ed. N. G. Haring and B. Bateman, 165–202.

Harste, J. C. 1985. Becoming a nation of language learners: Beyond risk. In *Toward Practical Theory: A State of Practice Assessment of Reading Comprehension Instruction. Final Report*, ed. J. C. Harste and D. Stevens, 8:1–122. Bloomington, IN: Indiana University.

Henk, W. A., Helfeldt, J. P., and Platt, J. M. 1986. Developing reading fluency in learning disabled students. *Teaching Exceptional Children* 12:202–6.

Henry, M. K. 1987. Understanding English orthography: Assessment instruction for decoding and spelling. Ph.D. diss., Stanford University, Palo Alto, CA.

Herr, C. M. 1984. Using Corrective Reading with adults. *Direct Instruction News*, Spring, 1984, 3–4.

Hillocks, G. 1984. What works in teaching composition: A meta-analysis of treatment studies. *American Journal of Education* 93:133–170.

Hinshelwood, J. 1917. *Congenital Word Blindness.* London: Lewis.

Hirsch, E., and Niedermeyer, F. C. 1973. The effects of tracing prompts and discrimination training on kindergarten handwriting performance. *Journal of Educational Research* 67:81–83.

Hiscock, M., and Kinsbourne, M. 1982. Laterality and dyslexia: A critical view. *Annals of Dyslexia* 32:177–228.

Hohn, W. F., and Ehri, L. C. 1983. Do alphabet letters help prereaders acquire phonemic segmentation skill? *Journal of Educational Psychology* 75:752–62.

Horn, E. 1960. Spelling. In *Encyclopedia for Educational Research,* ed. W. S. Monroe, 1337–54. New York: Macmillan.

Howard, M. 1982. Utilizing oral-motor feedback in auditory conceptualization. *Journal of Educational Neuropsychology* 2:24–35.

Howard, M. 1986. Effects of pre-reading training in auditory conceptualization on subsequent reading achievement. Ph.D. diss., Brigham Young University.

Hulme, C. 1981. *Reading Retardation and Multi-Sensory Teaching.* London: Routledge and Kegan Paul.

Inhelder, B., and Piaget, J. 1958. *The Growth of Logical Thinking from Childhood to Adolescence.* New York: Basic Books.

Inouye, D., and Sorenson, M. R. 1985. Profiles of disability: The computer as an instrument of vision. In *Biobehavioral Measures of Dyslexia,* ed. D. B. Gray and J. F. Kavanagh, 297–321. Parkton, MD: York Press.

Institute for Training and Research in Auditory Conceptualization (INTRAC). 1983. Santa Monica Preventive Study. San Luis Obispo, CA.

Jansky, J., and deHirsch, K. 1972. *Preventing Reading Failure: Prediction, Diagnosis, Intervention.* New York: Harper and Row.

Johnson, D. J., and Myklebust, H. R. 1967. *Learning Disabilities.* New York: Grune and Stratton.

Johnson, W. T. 1977. *The Johnson Handwriting Program.* Cambridge, MA: Educators Publishing Service.

Jorm, A. F., and Share, D. L. 1983. An invited article: Phonological recoding and reading acquisition. *Applied Psycholinguistics* 4:103–47.

Juel, C., Griffeth, P. L., and Gough, P. B. 1985. A longitudinal study of the changing relationships of word recognition, spelling, reading comprehension, and writing from first to second grade. Paper presented at the Annual Meeting of the American Educational Research Association, Chicago, April, 1985.

Just, M. A., and Carpenter, P. A. 1980. Theory of reading: From eye fixations to comprehension. *Psychological Review* 87:3329–54.

Karweit, N. 1985. Time spent, time needed, and adaptive instruction. In *Adapting Instruction to Individual Differences,* ed. M. C. Wang and H. I. Walberg, 281–97. Berkeley, CA: McCutchan.

Keogh, B. K., and Pelland, M. 1985. Vision training revisited. *Journal of Learning Disabilities* 18:228–36.

King, D. H. 1985. *Writing Skills for the Adolescent.* Cambridge, MA: Educators Publishing Service.

King, D. H. 1986. *Keyboarding Skills.* Cambridge, MA: Educators Publishing Service.

Kinsbourne, M., and Hiscock, M. 1981. Cerebral lateralization and cognitive development: Conceptual and methodological issues. In *Neuropsychological Assessment of the School-Age Child,* ed. G. W. Hynd and J. E. Obrzut, 125–66. New York: Grune and Stratton.

Kinsbourne, M., and Warrington, E. K. 1963. Developmental factors in reading and reading backwardness. *British Journal of Psychology* 54:145–56.

Kintsch, W., and van Dijk, T. A. 1978. Toward a model of text and comprehension production. *Psychological Review* 85:363–94.

Kirk, U. 1981. The development and use of rules in the acquisition of perceptual motor skills. *Child Development* 52:299–305.

Kleiman, G. M. 1975. Speech recoding and reading. *Journal of Verbal Learning and Verbal Behavior* 14:323–39.

Kline, C., and Kline, C. 1975. Follow-up study of 216 dyslexic children. *The Bulletin of The Orton Society* 25:127–44.

Knights, R. M. 1982. Computer-aided learning: Performance of hyperactive and learning disabled children. In *Theory and Research in Learning Disabilities,* ed. J. P. Das, R. F. Mulcahy, and A. E. Wall, 201–14. New York: Plenum Press.

LaBerge, D. 1979. The perception of units in beginning reading. In *Theory and Practice of Early Reading: Vol. 3,* ed. L. B. Resnick and P. A. Weaver, 31–51. Hillsdale, NJ: Lawrence Erlbaum Associates.

LaBerge, D., and Samuels, S. J. 1974. Toward a theory of automatic information processing in reading. *Cognitive Psychology* 6:293–323.

Leinhardt, G., Zigmond, N., and Cooley, W. W. 1980. Reading instruction and its effects. Paper presented at the Annual Meeting of the American Educational Research Association, April, 1980, Boston, MA.

Leong, C. K., and Enfield, M. L. 1986. Memo to Branch Council Presidents and National Board Members of The Orton Dyslexia Society, Jan. 15, 1986, Baltimore, MD.

Lesgold, A. M., and Resnick, L. B. 1982. How reading difficulties develop: Perspectives from a longitudinal study. In *Theory and Research in Learning Disabilities,* ed. R. F. Mulcahy and A. E. Wall, 155–88. New York: Plenum Press.

Lewkowicz, N. K. 1980. Phonemic awareness training: What to teach and how to teach it. *Journal of Educational Psychology* 72:686–700.

Liberman, I. Y. 1984. A language-directed view of reading and its disabilities. *Thalamus* 4: 1–41.

Liberman, I. Y., Liberman, A. M., Mattingly, I., and Shankweiler, D. 1983. Orthography and the beginning reader. In *Orthography, Reading, and Dyslexia,* ed. J. P. Kavanagh and R. L. Venezky, 137–53. Baltimore: University Park Press.

Liberman, I. Y., Mann, V. A., Shankweiler, D., and Werfelman, M. 1980. Children's memory for recurring linguistic and non-linguistic material in relation to reading ability. *Cortex* 18:367.

Liberman, I. Y., and Shankweiler, D. 1979. Speech, the alphabet, and teaching to read. In *Theory and Practice of Early Reading: Vol. 2,* ed. L. B. Resnick and P. A. Weaver, 109–32. Hillsdale, NJ: Lawrence Erlbaum Associates.

Liberman, I. Y., and Shankweiler, D. 1985. Phonology and the problems of learning to read and write. *Remedial and Special Education* 6:8–17.

Liberman, I. Y., Shankweiler, D., Fischer, F. W., and Carter, B. 1974. Explicit syllable and phoneme segmentation in the young child. *Journal of Experimental Child Psychology* 18:2-1–12.

Liberman, I. Y., Shankweiler, D., Liberman, A. M., Fowler, C., and Fischer, F. W. 1977. Phonetic segmentation and recoding in the beginning reader. In *Toward a Psychology of Reading,* ed. A. S. Rober and D. L. Scarborough, 207–25. Hillsdale, NJ: Lawrence Erlbaum Associates.

Lichenstein, R., and Ireton, H. 1984. *Preschool Screening.* New York: Grune and Stratton.

Lichter, J. H., and Roberge, L. P. 1979. First grade intervention for reading achievement of high risk children. *Bulletin of The Orton Society* 29:238–44.

Lindamood, C. H., and Lindamood, P. C. 1975. *The A.D.D. Program, Auditory Discrimination in Depth: Books 1 and 2.* Hingham, MA: Teaching Resources.

Lindamood, C. H., and Lindamood, P. C. 1979. *The LAC Test: Lindamood Auditory Conceptualization Test.* Allen, TX: DLM Teaching Resources.

Lindamood, P. C., and Lindamood, C. H. 1980. Diagnosing and remediating auditory conceptual dysfunction. *Proceedings of the 18th Congress of the International Association of Logopedics and Phoniatrics* 2:148–77.

Lipa, S. B. 1984. Reading disabilities: A new look at an old issue. *Annual Review of Learning Disabilities* 2:51–55.

Lipson, M. Y., and Wixson, K. K. 1986. Reading disability research: A new look at an old issue. *Review of Educational Research* 56:111–36.

Lloyd, J., Epstein, M. H., and Cullinan, D. 1981. Direct teaching for learning disabilities. In *Developmental Theory and Research in Learning Disabilities,* ed. J. Gottlieb and S. S. Strichart, 278–309. Baltimore: University Park Press.

Lorsbach, T. C., and Gray, J. W. 1985. Item identification speed and memory span performance in learning disabled children. Paper presented at the Annual Meeting of the American Educational Research Association, April, 1985, Chicago.

Lovett, M. W. 1984. The search for subtypes of specific reading disability: Reflections from a cognitive perspective. *Annals of Dyslexia* 34:155–78.

Lovitt, T. C., and DeMier, D. M. 1984. An evaluation of the Slingerland method with LD youngsters. *Journal of Learning Disabilities* 17:267–72.

Lundberg, I. 1985. Longitudinal studies of reading and reading difficulties in Sweden. In *Reading Research: Advances in Theory and Practice: Vol. 4,* ed. G. E. MacKinnon and T. G. Waller, 65–105. New York: Academic Press.

Lyon, G. R. 1985. Identification and remediation of learning disability subtypes: Preliminary findings. *Learning Disabilities Focus* 1:21–35.

McKeown, M. G., and Beck, I. L. 1988. Learning vocabulary: Different ways for different goals. *Remedial and Special Education* 9:42–46.

MacArthur, C. A., and Graham, S. 1988. Learning disabled students composing under three methods of text production: Handwriting, word processing, and dictation. *The Journal of Special Education* 21:22–42.

MacArthur, C. A., and Shneiderman, B. 1986. Learning disabled students' difficulties in learning to use a word processor: Implications for instruction and software evaluation. *Journal of Learning Disabilities* 19:248–53.

Mann, V. A. 1984. Longitudinal prediction and prevention of early reading difficulty. *Annals of Dyslexia* 34:117–56.

Mann, V. A. 1986. Why some children encounter reading problems: The contribution of difficulties with language processing and phonological sophistication to early reading disability. In *Psychological and Educational Perspectives on Learning Disabilities,* ed. J. K. Torgeson and B. Y. L. Wong, 133–59. New York: Academic Press.

Mann, V. A., and Liberman, I. Y. 1984. Phonological awareness and verbal short-term memory. *Journal of Learning Disabilities* 17:592–99.

Mann, V. A., Shankweiler, D., and Smith, S. 1984. The association between comprehension of spoken sentences and early reading ability: The role of phonetic representation. *Journal of Child Language* 11:627–43.

Maria, K. 1986. Adapting the new comprehension techniques for the learning disabled child. Paper presented to the Thirteenth Annual Conference of the N. Y. Branch of The Orton Dyslexia Society, March, 1986, New York.

Maria, K., and MacGinitie, W. H. 1982. Reading comprehension disabilities: Knowledge structures and non-accommodating text processing strategies. *Annals of Dyslexia* 32:33–59.

Markowsky, M. E. 1987. The effects of an oral language supplement on Writing to Read for at risk and average kindergarten children. Ed.D. diss., Teachers College, Columbia University, New York.

Martin, J. H. 1985. The Writing to Read system and reading difficulties: Some preliminary observations. In *Understanding Learning Disabilities,* ed.D. D. Duane and C. K. Leong, 159–63. New York: Plenum Press.

Martin, J. H., and Friedberg, A. 1986. *Writing to Read.* New York: Warner Books.

Mattingly, I. G. 1972. Reading, the linguistic process, and linguistic awareness. In *Language by Ear and by Eye: The Relationship between Speech and Reading,* ed. J. F. Kavanagh and I. G. Mattingly, 133–48. Cambridge, MA: MIT Press.

Mattis, S., French, J. H., and Rapin, I. 1975. Dyslexia in children and young adults: Three independent neuropsychological syndromes. *Developmental Medicine and Child Neurology* 17:150–63.

McCulloch, C. 1985. The Slingerland approach: Is it effective in a specific language disability classroom? M.A. thesis, Seattle Pacific University, Seattle, WA.

Menynuk, P., and Flood, J. 1981. Linguistic competence, reading, writing problems, and remediation. *Bulletin of The Orton Society* 31:13–28.

Metzger, R. L., and Werner, D. B. 1984. Use of visual training for reading disabilities: A review. *Pediatrics* 73:824–29.

Meyer, L. A. 1984. Long-term academic effects of the direct instruction project Follow-Through. *Elementary School Journal* 84:380–94.

Meyer, L. A., Gersten, R. M., and Gutkin, J. 1983. Direct Instruction: A Project Follow-Through success story in an inner-city school. *Elementary School Journal* 84:241–52.

Moats, L. C. 1983. A comparison of the spelling errors of older dyslexic and second grade normal children. *Annals of Dyslexia* 33:121–39.

Mokros, J. R., and Russell, S. J. 1986. Learner-centered software: A survey of microcomputer use with special needs students. *Journal of Learning Disabilities* 19:185–90.

Montessori, M. 1964. *The Montessori Method.* New York: Schocken Books.

Moore, M. J., Kagan, J., Sahl, M., and Grant, S. 1982. Cognitive profiles in reading disabilities. *Genetic Psychology Monographs* 105:41–93.

Morais, J., Cary, L., Algeria, J., and Bertelson, P. 1979. Does awareness of speech as a sequence of phonemes arise spontaneously? *Cognition* 7:323–31.

Morocco, C. C., and Neuman, S. B. 1986. Word processors and the acquisition of writing strategies. *Journal of Learning Disabilities* 19:243–47.

Murphy, R. T., and Appel, L. R. 1984. *Evaluation of the Writing to Read Instructional System.* Princeton, NJ: Educational Testing Service.

Myklebust, H. R. 1965, *Development and Disorders of Written Language: Vol. 1. Picture Story Language Test.* New York: Grune and Stratton.

Myklebust, H. R., and Johnson, D. J. 1962. Dyslexia in children. *Exceptional Children* 29:14–25.

Nelson, H. E., and Warrington, E. K. 1980. An investigation of memory functions in dyslexic children. *British Journal of Psychology* 71:487–503.

Nockleby, D. M., and Galbraith, G. G. 1984. Developmental dyslexia subtypes and the Boder Test of Reading-Spelling Patterns. *Journal of Psychoeducational Assessment* 2:91–100.

Obrzut, J. E., and Boliek, C. A. 1986. Lateralization characteristics in learning disabled children. *Journal of Learning Disabilities* 19:308–14.

Olson, R. K., Kliegl, R., Davidson, B. J., and Folz, G. 1985. Individual and developmental differences in reading disability. In *Reading Research: Advances in Theory and Practice: Vol. 4,* ed. C. E. MacKinnon and T. G. Waller, 1–63. New York: Academic Press.

Orton, J. 1964. *A Guide to Teaching Phonics.* Cambridge, MA: Educators Publishing Service.

Orton, J. 1966. The Orton-Gillingham approach. In *The Disabled Reader,* ed. J. Money, 119–46. Baltimore: The Johns Hopkins University Press.

Orton, S. T. 1925. Word-blindness in school children. *Archives of Neurology and Psychology* 14:581–615.

Orton, S. T. 1937. *Reading, Writing, and Speech Problems in Children.* New York: Norton.

Otto, W., Wolf, A., and Eldridge, R. G. 1984. Managing instruction. In *Handbook of Reading Research,* ed. P. D. Pearson, 799–828. New York: Longman.

Palinscar, A., and Brown, A. 1983. Reciprocal teaching of comprehension-monitoring activities (Technical Report No. 269). Urbana, Il: The University of Illinois, Center for the Study of Reading.

Palinscar, A., and Brown, A. 1985. Reciprocal teaching: A means to a meaningful end. In *Reading Education: Foundations for a Literate America,* ed. J. Osborn, P. T. Wilson, and R. C. Anderson, 199–310. Lexington, MA: D. C. Heath.

Pavlidis, G. T. 1985. Eye movements in dyslexia: Their diagnostic significance. *Journal of Learning Disabilities* 18:42–50.

Pearson, P. D. 1982. A context for instructional research on reading comprehension (Technical Report No. 230). Urbana, Il: University of Illinois, Center for the Study of Reading.

Pearson, P. D., and Gallagher, M. C. 1983. The instruction of reading comprehension. *Contemporary Educational Psychology;* 8:317–44.

Pearson, P. D., and Leys, M. 1985. "Teaching" comprehension. In *Reading, Thinking, and Concept Development,* ed. T. L. Harris and E. J. Cooper, 3–20. New York: College Board Publications.

Peister, P., Fadiman, S., Pierce, K., and Fayne, H. 1978–1980. Integrative review of basic reading skills. *Integrative Reviews of Research: Vol. 1,* 71–134. New York: Teachers College, Institute for the Study of Learning Disabilities.

Pennington, B. F., Lefly, D. L., Van Orden, G. C., Bookman, M. O., and Smith, S. D. 1987. Is phonology bypassed in normal or dyslexic development? *Annals of Dyslexia* 37:62–89.

Perfetti, C. A. 1984. Reading acquisition and beyond: Decoding includes cognition. *American Journal of Education* 93:40–60.

Perfetti, C. A. 1985a. Continuities in reading acquisition, reading skills, and reading disability. *Remedial and Special Education* 7:11–21.

Perfetti, C. A. 1985b. *Reading Ability.* New York: Oxford University Press.

Perfetti, C. A., and Hogaboam, T. 1975. Relationship between single word decoding and reading comprehension skill. *Journal of Educational Psychology* 67:461–69.

Perfetti, C. A., and Lesgold, A. M. 1979. Coding and comprehension in skilled reading and implications for reading instruction. In *Theory and Practice of Early Reading: Vol. 1,* ed. L. B. Resnick and P. A. Weaver, 57–84. Hillsdale, NJ: Lawrence Erlbaum Associates.

Perfetti, C. A., and Roth, S. 1981. Some of the interactive processes in reading and their role in reading skill. In *Interactive Processes in Reading,* ed. A. M. Lesgold and C. A. Perfetti, 269–97. Hillsdale, NJ: Lawrence Erlbaum Associates.

Petrauskas, R., and Rourke, B. 1979. Identification of subgroups of retarded readers: A neuropsychological multivariate approach. *Journal of Clinical Neuropsychology* 1:17–37.

Pflaum, S. W., Walberg, H. J., Karegianes, M. L., and Rasher, P. 1980. Reading instruction: A quantitative analysis. *Educational Researcher* 9:12–18.

Phelps, J., and Stempel, L. 1987. Handwriting: Evolution and evaluation. *Annals of Dyslexia* 37:228–39.

Piaget, J. 1970. *Structuralism.* New York: Basic Books.

Poe, L. B. 1983. The effects of a supplemental intervention training program on first graders who lack segmentation ability. Ed.D. diss., University of Southern Mississippi, Hattiesburg, MS.

Polloway, E. A., and Epstein, M. H. 1986. The use of Corrective Reading (SRA) with mildly handicapped students. *Direct Instruction News,* 2–3.

Poplin, M. 1983. Assessing developmental writing abilities. *Topics in Learning and Learning Disabilities* 3:63–75.

Poplin, M., Gray, R., Larsen, S., Banikowski, A., and Mehring, T. 1980. A comparison of components of written expression abilities in learning disabled and non-disabled students at three grade levels. *Learning Disability Quarterly* 3:46–59.

Poteet, J. 1980. Informal assessment of written expression. *Learning Disability Quarterly* 3: 88–98.

Punnet, A. F., and Steinhauer, G. D. 1984. Relationship between reinforcement and eye movements during ocular motor training with learning disabled children. *Journal of Learning Disabilities* 17:16–20.

Rashotte, C. A. 1983. Repeated reading and reading fluency in learning disabled children. Ph.D. diss., The Florida State University, Tallahassee, FL.

Rashotte, C. A., and Torgesen, J. K. 1985. Repeated reading and reading fluency in learning disabled children. *Reading Research Quarterly* 20:180–88.

Rasmussen, D. E., and Goldberg, L. 1976. *SRA Basic Reading.* Chicago, IL: Science Research Associates.

Raynor, K. 1985. The role of eye movements in learning to read and reading disability. *Remedial and Special Education* 6:53–60.

Read, C. 1970. Children's perceptions of the sounds of English phonology from three to six. Ph.D. diss., Harvard Graduate School of Education, Cambridge, MA.

Read, C. 1975. Lessons to be learned from the preschool orthographer. In *Foundations of Language Development: Vol. 2,* ed. E. H. Lennenberg and E. Lennenberg, 329–46. New York: Academic Press.

Read, C., and Ruyter, L. 1985. Reading and spelling skills in adults of low literacy. *Remedial and Special Education* 6:43–52.

Reid, E. 1986. Practicing effective instruction: The Exemplary Center for Reading Instruction approach. *Exceptional Children* 52:510–519.

Resnick, L. B. 1979. Theories and prescriptions for early reading. In *Theory and Practice of Early Reading: Vol. 2,* ed. L. G. Resnick and P. A. Weaver, 321–28. Hillsdale, NJ: Lawrence Erlbaum Associates.

Richardson, E., and DiBenedetto, B. 1985. *The Decoding Skills Test.* Parkton, MD: York Press.

Richardson, E., DiBenedetto, B., and Adler, A. 1982. Use of the Decoding Skills Test to study the differences between good and poor readers. In *Advances in Learning and Behavioral Disabilities,* ed. K. D. Gadow and I. Bialer, 25–74. Greenwich, CT: JAI Press.

Robinson, H. 1972. Visual and auditory modalities related to methods for beginning reading. *Reading Research Quarterly* 8:7–39.

Robinson, H., and Schwartz, L. B.. 1973. Visuo-motor skills and reading ability: A longitudinal study. *Developmental Medicine and Child Neurology* 15:281–86.

Rosenshine, B. 1983. Teaching functions in instructional programs. *Elementary School Journal* 83:335–340.

Rosenshine, B., and Stevens, R. 1984. Classroom instruction in reading. In *Handbook of Reading Research,* ed. P. D. Pearson, 745–98. New York: Longman.

Rosner, J. 1974. Auditory analysis training with prereaders. *The Reading Teacher* 27:379–81.

Rosner, J. 1975. *Helping Children Overcome Learning Disabilities.* New York: Walker and Company.

Rosner, J., and Simon, D. P. 1971. The auditory analysis test: An initial report. *Journal of Learning Disabilities* 4:384–92.

Roth, S., and Beck, I. 1984. Research and instructional issues related to the enhancement of children's decoding skills through two microcomputer programs. Paper presented at the Annual Meeting of the American Educational Research Association, April, 1984, New Orleans.

Roy, B. J. 1986. A cooperative teacher education and language retraining program for dyslexics in West Texas. Paper presented at the Action in Research V, Conference, Jan., 1986. Lubbock, TX.

Rumelhart, D. E. 1977. Toward an interactive model of reading. In *Attention and Performance VI,* ed., S. Dornic, 45–67. Hillsdale, NJ: Lawrence Erlbaum Associates.

Rumelhart, D. E. 1980. Schemata: The building blocks of cognition. In *Theoretical Issues in Reading Comprehension,* ed. R. J. Spiro, B. C. Bruce, and W. F. Brewer, 33–58. Hillsdale, NJ: Lawrence Erlbaum Associates.

Rutter, M. 1978. The prevalence and types of dyslexia. *Dyslexia: An Appraisal of Current Knowledge,* ed. A. L. Benton and D. Pearl, 5–28. New York: Oxford University Press.

Ryan, M. C., Miller, C. E., and Witt, J. C. 1984. A comparison of the use of orthographic structure in word discrimination by learning disabled and normal children. *Journal of Learning Disabilities* 17:38–40.

Samuels, S. J. 1979. The method of repeated readings. *The Reading Teacher* 32:402–8.

Samuels, S. J. 1986. Automaticity and repeated readings. In *Reading Education: Foundations for a Literate America,* ed. J. Osborn, P. T. Wilson, and R. C. Anderson, 215–30. Lexington, MA: D. C. Heath.

Satz, P., and Morris, R. 1980. Learning disability subtypes: A review. In *Neuropsychological and Cognitive Processing in Reading,* ed. F. J. Pirrozolo and M. C. Wittrock, 124–135. New York: Academic Press.

Satz, P., Saslow, E., and Henry, R. 1985. The pathological left-handedness syndrome. *Brain and Cognition* 4:27–46.

Scarborough, H. S. 1984. Continuity between childhood dyslexia and adult reading. *British Journal of Psychology* 75:329–348.

Schreiber, P. A. 1980. On the acquisition of reading fluency. *Journal of Reading Behavior* 12:177–86.

Shanahan, T. 1984. The nature of the reading-writing relationship: An exploratory multivariate analysis. *Journal of Educational Psychology* 76:466–77.

Shanahan, T., and Lomax, R. 1985. An analysis and comparison of theoretical models of the reading-writing relationship. Paper presented at the Annual Meeting of the American Educational Research Association, April, 1985, Chicago.

Shucard, D. W., Cummins, K. R., Gay, E., Lairsmith, J., and Welanko, P. 1985. Electrophysiological studies of reading disabled children: In search of subtypes. *Biobehavioral Measures of Dyslexia,* ed. D. B. Gray and J. F. Kavanagh, 87–106. Parkton, MD: York Press.

Siegel, L. 1985. Psycholinguistic aspects of reading disabilities. In *Cognitive Development of Atypical Children,* ed. L. S. Siegel and F. J. Morrison, 45–65. New York: Springer Verlag.

Silverman, R., Zigmond, N., Zimmerman, J. M., and Vallescorsa, B. 1981. Improving written expression in learning disabled adolescents. *Journal of Learning Disabilities* 16:478–82.

Slingerland, B. H. 1971. *A Multi-Sensory Approach to Language Arts for Specific Language Disability Children: A Guide for Primary Teachers, Books 1–3.* Cambridge, MA: Educators Publishing Service.

Slingerland, B. H. 1976. *Basics in Scope and Sequence of a Multi-Sensory Approach to Language Arts for SLD Children.* Cambridge, MA: Educators Publishing Service.

Smiley, S., Oakley, D., Worthern, D., Campione, J., and Brown, A. 1977. Recall of thematically relevant material by adolescent good and poor readers as a function of written versus oral presentation. *Journal of Educational Psychology* 69:381–87.

Smith, F. 1978. *Understanding Reading: A Psycholinguistic Analysis of Reading and Learning to Read.* New York: Holt, Rinehart, and Winston.

Smith, F. 1979. Conflicting approaches to reading research and instruction. In *Theory and Practice of Early Reading: Vol. 2,* ed. L. B. Resnick and P. A. Weaver, 31–42. Hillsdale, NJ: Lawrence Erlbaum Associates.

Spalding, R. B., and Spalding, W. T. 1986. *The Writing Road to Reading.* New York: Quill/William Morrow.

Stanback, M., and Hansen, M. 1980. Integrative review of spelling. In *Integrative Reviews of Research: Vol 1,* 135–200. New York: Teachers College, Institute for the Study of Learning Disabilities.

Stanovich, K. E. 1980. Toward an interactive-compensatory model of individual differences in the development of reading fluency. *Reading Research Quarterly* 1:32–7.

Stanovich, K. E. 1984. The interactive-compensatory model of reading: A confluence of developmental, experimental, and educational psychology. *Remedial and Special Education* 5:11–19.

Stanovich, K. E. 1985. Explaining the variance in reading ability in terms of psychological processes: What have we learned? *Annals of Dyslexia* 35:67–95.

Stanovich, K. E. 1986a. Cognitive processes and the reading problems of learning disabled children: Evaluating the assumption of specificity. In *Psychological and Educational Perspectives on Learning Disabilities,* ed. J. K. Torgesen and B. Y. L. Wong, 87–131. New York: Academic Press.

Stanovich, K. E. 1986b. Matthew effects in reading: Some consequences of individual differences in the acquisition of literacy. *Reading Research Quarterly* 21:360–407.

Stanovich, K. E., Cunningham, A. E., and Cramer, B. B. 1984. Assessing phonological awareness in kindergarten children: issues of task comparability. *Journal of Experimental Child Psychology* 38:1–90.

Stanovich, K. E., Cunningham, A. E., and Feeman, D. J. 1984. Intelligence, cognitive skills, and early reading progress. *Reading Research Quarterly* 29:278–303.

Stark, R. E., Bernstein, L. E., Condino, R., Bender, M., Tallal, P., and Catts, H. 1984. Four-year follow-up study of language impaired children. *Annals of Dyslexia* 34:49–68.

Steeves, K. J. 1987. The use of computers in the education of the dyslexic child. Paper presented at the Fourteenth Annual Conference of the New York Branch of The Orton Dyslexia Society, March, 1987, New York.

Steffenson, M. S., Joag-Dev, C., and Anderson, R. C. 1979. A cross-cultural perspective on reading comprehension. *Reading Research Quarterly* 15:10–29.

Stephens, D. 1985. Uncharted land: Reading comprehension research with the special education student. In *Landscapes: A State-of-the-Art Assessment of Reading Comprehension Research, 1974–1984: Vol. 1,* ed. A. Crismore, 5:1–5:19. Bloomington, IN: Indiana University.

Stern, C., and Gould, T. 1965. *Children Discover Reading.* New York: Random House.

Strominger, A. Z., and Bashir, A. S. 1977. Longitudinal study of language-delayed children. Paper presented at the Annual Convention of the American Speech and Hearing Association.

Strother, M. E. 1984. Effects of automaticity training strategies on word recognition. Ph.D. diss., Arizona State University, Tempe, AZ.

Tallal, P. 1980. Language and reading: Some perceptual prerequisites. *Bulletin of The Orton Society* 30:170–78.

Tallal, P., and Stark, R. E. 1982. Perceptual/motor profiles of reading impaired children with or without concomitant oral language deficits. *Annals of Dyslexia* 32:163–76.

Tharp, R. G. 1982. The effective instruction of comprehension: Results and description of the Kamehameha Early Education Program. *Reading Research Quarterly* 17:503–27.

Thorndyke, P. W., and Hayes-Roth, B. 1979. The use of schemata in the acquisition and transfer of knowledge. *Cognitive Psychology* 11 2–106.

Tierney, R. J., and Cunningham, J. W. 1984. Research on teaching reading comprehension. In *Handbook of Reading Research,* ed. P. D. Pearson, 609–56. New York: Longman.

Torgesen, J.K. 1985. Memory processes in reading disabled children. *Journal of Learning Disabilities* 18:350–57.

Torgesen, J. K., and Young, K. A. 1984. Priorities for the use of microcomputer with learning disabled children. *Annual Review of Learning Disabilities* 2:143–46.

Traub, N. 1982. Reading, spelling, handwriting: Traub Systematic Holistic Method. *Annals of Dyslexia* 32:135–45.

Traub, N., and Bloom, F. 1975. *Recipe for Reading*. Cambridge, MA: Educators Publishing Service.

Treiman, R., and Baron, J. 1983. Individual differences in spelling: The Phoenician-Chinese distinction. *Topics in Learning Disabilities* 3:33–40.

Turner, S., and Dawson, M. 1978. The teaching of reading: A review. *Journal of Learning Disabilities* 11:17–27.

Vellutino, F. 1978. Toward an understanding of dyslexia: Psychological factors in specific reading disability. In *Dyslexia: An Appraisal of Current Knowledge,* ed. A. L. Benton and D. Pearl, 163–71. New York: Oxford University Press.

Vellutino, F. 1983. Dyslexia; Perceptual deficiency of perceptual inefficiency. In *Orthography, Reading, and Dyslexia,* ed. J. P. Kavanagh and R. L. Venezky, 251–69. Baltimore: University Park Press.

Vellutino, F. 1987. Dyslexia. *Scientific American* 256(3):34–41.

Vellutino, F., and Scanlon, D. M. 1986. Experimental evidence for the effects of instructional bias on word identification. *Exceptional Children* 53:145–56.

Vellutino, F., Steger, J. A., Kaman, M., and DeSetto, L. 1975. Visual form perception in deficient and normal readers as a function of age and orthographic linguistic familiarity. *Cortex* 11:22–30.

Vellutino, F., Steger, J. A., and Kandel, G. 1972. Reading disability: An investigation of the perceptual deficit hypothesis. *Cortex* 8:106–18.

Vellutino, F., Steger, J. A., and Pruzek, R. 1973. Inter- vs. intrasensory deficit in paired associate learning in poor and normal readers. *Canadian Journal of Behavioral Science* 5:111–23.

Venezky, R. L. 1970. *The Structure of English Orthography*. The Hague, Holland: Moulton.

Venezky, R. L. 1976. Prerequisites for learning to read. In *Cognitive Learning in Children: Theories and Strategies,* ed. R. Levin and V. L. Allen, 163–85. New York: Academic Press.

Venezky, R. L., and Massaro, D. W. 1979. The role of orthographic regularity in word recognition. In *Theory and Practice of Early Reading: Vol. 1,* ed. L. B. Resnick and P. A. Weaver, 85–107. Hillsdale, NJ: Lawrence Erlbaum Associates.

Vickery, K. S., Reynolds, V. A., and Cochran, S. W. 1987. Multisensory teaching for reading, spelling, and handwriting, Orton-Gillingham based, in a public school setting. *Annals of Dyslexia* 37:189–202.

Vogel, S. A. 1975. *Syntactic Abilities in Normal and Dyslexic Children*. Baltimore: University Park Press.

Vygotsky, L. S. 1978. *Mind in Society,* ed. and trans. M. Cole, V. John-Steiner, S. Scribner, and E. Souberman. Cambridge, MA: Harvard University Press.

Wagner, R. K., and Torgesen, J. K. 1987. The nature of phonological processing and its causal role in the acquisition of reading skills. *Psychological Bulletin* 101:192–212.

Wallach, M. A., and Wallach, L. 1979. Helping disadvantaged children learn to read by teaching them phoneme identification skills. In *Theory and Practice of Early Reading: Vol. 3,* 197–215. Hillsdale, NJ: Lawrence Erlbaum Associates.

Webster's Third New International Dictionary of the English Language Unabridged. 1976. Springfield, MA: G. and C. Merriam Company.

Weiner, M. J. 1980. Diagnostic evaluation of writing skills. *Journal of Learning Disabilities* 1:48–53.

Williams, J. P. 1975. Training children to copy and discriminate letter like forms. *Journal of Educational Psychology* 67:790–95.

Williams, J. P. 1980. Teaching decoding with an emphasis on phoneme analysis and phoneme blending. *Journal of Experimental Psychology* 72:1–15.

Williams, J. P. 1985. The case for explicit decoding instruction. In *Reading Education: Foundations for a Literate America,* ed. J. Osborn, P. T. Wilson, and R. C. Anderson, 205–13. Lexington, MA: D. C. Heath.

Williams, J. P. 1986a. The role of phonemic analysis in reading. In *Psychological and Educational Perspectives on Learning Disabilities,* Ed. J. K. Torgesen and B. Y. L. Wong, 399–416. New York: Academic Press.

Williams, J. P. 1986b. Teaching children to identify the main idea of expository texts. *Exceptional Children* 53:163–68.

Wolf, B. J. 1985. The effect of Slingerland instruction on the reading and language of second grade children. Ph.D. diss., Seattle Pacific University, Seattle, WA.

Wolf, M. 1984. Naming, reading, and the dyslexias: A longitudinal overview. *Annals of Dyslexia* 34:87–115.

Wolff, D. E., Desberg, P., and Marsh, G. 1985. Analogy strategies for improving word recognition in competent learning disabled readers. *The Reading Teacher* 38:412–16.

Wright, D. C., and Wright, J. P. 1980. Handwriting: The effectiveness of copying from moving vs. still models. *Journal of Educational Research* 74:95–8.

Yee, A. H. 1966. The generalization controversy on spelling instruction. *Elementary English* 43:154–63.

Ysseldyke, J. E., and Algozzine, B. 1983. Where to begin in diagnosing reading problems. *Topics in Learning and Learning Disabilities* 2:60–9.

Zaner-Bloser. 1987. *Zaner-Bloser Handwriting: Basic Skills and Application, K–8*. Columbus, OH: Zaner-Bloser.

Zigmond, N. 1966. Intrasensory and intersensory processes in normal and dyslexic children. Ph.D. diss., Northwestern University, Chicago.

Zigmond, N., and Miller, S. E.. 1986. Assessment for instructional planning. *Exceptional Children* 52:501–9.

Zigmond, N., and Thornton, H. 1985. Follow-up of postsecondary age learning disabled graduates and drop-outs. *Learning Disabilities Research* 1:50–5.

Resource and Teacher Training Guide

The Aylett Royall Cox Institute
4111 North Central Expressway, Suite 201
Dallas, Texas 75204-2197
Tel. 214-521-7622

The Neuhaus Education Center
3131 West Alabama Street, Suite 208
Houston, Texas 77098
Tel. 713-520-6860

The Katheryne B. Payne Foundation
900 Northwest 10th Street
Oklahoma City, Oklahoma 73106
Tel. 405-236-1512

The Alphabetic Phonics Institute
Box 223, Department of Special Education
Teachers College, Columbia University
525 West 125th Street
New York, NY 10027
Tel. 212-678-3080

Lena W. Waters Memorial Teacher Training Program
Scottish Rite Learning Center of West Texas
602 Avenue Q
Lubbock, Texas 79401
Tel. 806-765-9150

ALPHABETIC PHONICS ADAPTATIONS

DYSLEXIA TRAINING PROGRAM

Child Development Division, Dyslexia Laboratory
Scottish Rite Hospital for Crippled Children
2222 Welborn Street
Dallas, Texas 75219
Tel. 214-521-3168

MULTISENSORY TEACHING APPROACH (MTA)

Edmar Educational Services
9550 Forest Lane, Suite 410
Dallas, Texas 75243
Tel. 214-503-1500

DISTAR AND CORRECTIVE READING

Association for Direct Instruction
P.O. Box 110252
Eugene, Oregon 97440
Tel. 503-485-1293

LINDAMOOD'S AUDITORY DISCRIMINATION IN DEPTH

Lindamood-Bell Learning Processes
416 Higuera Street
San Luis Obispo, California 93401
Tel. 805-489-2823

THE ORTON-GILLINGHAM APPROACH

The Carroll School
Baker Bridge Road
Lincoln, Massachusetts 01773
Tel. 617-259-8342

Language Disorders Unit
A.C.C. Massachusetts General Hospital
Boston, Massachusetts 02114
Tel. 617-726-2764

Michigan Dyslexia Institute
Decoding and Encoding Seminars
2356 Science Parkway, Suite 100
Okemos, Michigan 48864
Tel. 1-800-832-3535

Pine Ridge School
1075 Williston Road
Williston, Vermont 05495
Tel. 802-434-2161

The Reading Center
622 5th Street, S.W.
Rochester, Minnesota 55902
Tel. 507-288-5217

PROJECT READ (CALFEE)

Calfee Project: Project READ
School of Education
Stanford University

PROJECT READ (ENFIELD AND GREENE)

% The Language Circle
P.O. Box 20631
Bloomington, Minnesota 55420
Tel. 612-887-9168

RECIPE FOR READING

% Mrs. Connie Russo
323 Concord Street
Dix Hills, New York 11746
Tel. 516-242-8943

THE SLINGERLAND MULTI-SENSORY APPROACH TO LANGUAGE ARTS

The Slingerland Institute
1 Bellevue Center
411 198th Avenue, N.E.
Bellevue, Washington 98004
Tel. 206-453-1190

WRITING TO READ

Information on program implementation and teacher training for this program can be obtained at local IBM branch offices.

ADDITIONAL RESOURCE

The Orton Dyslexia Society
International Headquarters
724 York Road
Baltimore, Maryland 21204
Tel. 301-296-0232

This is an extremely useful resource for parents as well as teachers of dyslexic students. The organization has branches in many areas throughout
the country.

Glossary of Terms

Affix—a letter or group of letters attached to the beginning or ending of a base word which changes the meaning of that word.

Allomorph—one of two or more forms of the same morpheme (see definition of morpheme).

Digraph—two successive letters in the same syllable representing a single speech sound.

    a. *Consonant digraph*—two successive letters representing a single consonant sound, e.g., *sh*.

    b. *Vowel digraph*—two successive letters representing a single vowel sound, e.g., *ai* (Cox 1984, p. 15)

Diphthong—two adjacent vowels in the same syllable whose sounds blend together. There are four diphthongs in English: *ou,* as in "out"; *ow,* as in "cow", *oi,* as in "oil", and *oy,* as in "boy" (Cox 1984, p. 15).

Dysgraphia—severe handwriting disorder due to poor eye-hand coordination.

Etymology—the study of the origins and derivations of words.

Gestalt—a pattern or configuration which constitutes, and is conceived as, a unit or whole.

Grapheme—a single letter or letter cluster representing a single speech sound (Cox 1984, 17).

Inflectional ending—a morpheme added to the end of a word which changes its meaning in terms of grammatical case, number, gender, or tense. Examples: *ing* in "ending"; *ed* in "ended"; *s* in "dogs"; *'s* in "dog's."

Laterality—the choice of hand, eye, or foot in performing everyday activities.

Lateralization—dominance of one or the other cerebral hemisphere for any form of brain functioning.

Lexicon—a body of word knowledge.

Morpheme—a meaningful unit of speech. A morpheme may be a whole word, e.g., *child;* a base word, e.g., *child* in "childhood"; a suffix, e.g., *hood* in "childhood"; or a prefix, e.g., *un* in "untie." A single morpheme may have many forms, as for example, the morpheme for plurality: *s* in "dogs," *es* in "foxes," *en* in "children," *i* in "foci," *a* in "data," *ae* in "alumnae." Each of these forms is an *allomorph* of the morpheme for plurality.

Morphograph—written form of a word part that has meaning, such as the ending *tion.*

Morphological—in linguistic terms, an adjective referring to meaningful units of speech; a suffix, for example, is a morphological (or inflectional) ending.

Multisensory—involving three or more human senses, usually visual, auditory, and kinesthetic.

Neuron—a nerve cell.

Orthography—the spelling of written language.

Orthographic—pertaining to the spelling of written language.

Phoneme—an individual sound unit in spoken words. The "smallest unit of speech that distinguishes one utterance from another . . . in the speech of a particular person or particular dialect. . . . " (Webster's Third, 1700).

Phonetic—pertaining to "speech sounds and their relation to graphic or written symbols" (Cox 1984, 24).

Phonetics—"The study and systematic classification of sounds made in spoken utterance. . . . " (Webster's Third, 1700).

Phonics—1. "The science of sound" (Webster's Third, 1700). 2. "The central use of letter-sound connections in the teaching of reading and spelling" (Cox 1984, 25).

Phonogram—"A symbol or symbols used to represent a single speech sound" (Cox 1984, 25).

Phonological—pertaining to the speech sounds in words.

Phonology—the science of speech sounds, including the development of speech sounds in one language or comparison of speech sound development in different languages (Webster's Third, 1700).

Prefix—a morpheme (letter or combination of letters) attached to the beginning of a base word which changes the meaning of that word.

Schema—in psychological terms, a theoretical framework of knowledge. Plural form: schemata.

Schwa—an unaccented vowel whose pronunciation approximates short *u*, as the first and last *a* in "America" or the *o* in "carrot".

Suffix—a morpheme (letter or combination of letters) attached to the end of a word which changes the meaning of that word.

Syntax—sentence structure. "That part of grammar which treats the relation of words, according to established usage" (Cox 1984, 31).

Index